Student Workbook

to Accompany

Pearson's Comprehensive
Medical Coding
A Path to Success

Jennifer Lame

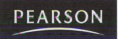

PEARSON

Boston   Columbus   Indianapolis   New York   San Francisco
Amsterdam   Cape Town   Dubai   London   Madrid   Milan   Munich   Paris   Montreal   Toronto
Delhi   Mexico City   São Paulo   Sydney   Hong Kong   Seoul   Singapore   Taipei   Tokyo

Publisher: Julie Levin Alexander
Publisher's Assistant: Regina Bruno
Acquisitions Editor: Marlene Pratt
Editorial Assistant: Lauren Bonilla
Program Manager: Faye Gemmellaro
Project Manager: Yagnesh Jani
Program Management, Team Lead: Melissa Bashe
Project Mangagement, Team Lead: Cindy Zonneveld
Marketing Manager: Brittany Hammond
Senior Marketing Coordinator: Alicia Wozniak
Marketing Specialist: Michael Sirinides
Full-Service Project Management: Amy L. Saucier, SPi Laserwords
Senior Operations Specialist: Mary Ann Gloriande
Media Project Manager: William Johnson
Creative Director: Andrea Nix
Art Director: Maria Guglielmo-Walsh
Composition: SPi Laserwords
Printing and Binding: Edwards Brothers Malloy
Cover Printer: Edwards Brothers Malloy

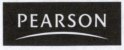

www.pearsonhighered.com

ISBN 0-13-380021-0
ISBN 978-0-13-380021-0

CONTENTS

PREFACE

This workbook is designed to accompany the textbook *Pearson's Comprehensive Medical Coding*.

Many of its features will allow you to work at your own pace and help you evaluate your progress throughout the course. Answers are provided in an answer key located within the Instructor's Resource Manual. There are features that will present a number of different ways to assess your progress as you journey through the text. Types of assessment features include:

Scavenger Hunt—These are included in each chapter and include activities to help you further explore topics presented in the textbook and how these relate to the professional world of coding.

Application Assignment—This section asks you to review a coding concept or process in more detail and reflect on how this information will benefit you in your future coding career.

Critical Thinking Assignment—This feature helps you master the Official Coding Guidelines by exploring these more in depth and how these apply to each chapter.

Chapter Review Questions:—These questions serve as a nice feature to review key concepts discussed in a chapter.

Interview with a Coder—In this activity you will be able to speak with a current coding professional about the role of a coder, the work setting, challenges and what a typical day is like.

Anatomy Labeling—In some chapters, you are asked to identify anatomic structures and/or color a blank image with the appropriate structures.

Coding Cases—This feature will reinforce your understanding of how to abstract out diagnoses and procedures from medical record documentation and apply the Official Coding Guidelines to these as you assign the correct codes.

We hope this workbook helps make your journey through comprehensive coding an enjoyable one.

Chapter

1

SCAVENGER HUNT

Research Professional Organizations

Two coding professional organizations are widely known and accepted as industry experts. These two organizations are the American Health Information Management Association (AHIMA) and the American Academy of Professional Coders (AAPC). Go to each website www.ahima.org and www.aapc.com and review each organization. The members, offerings for members, benefits of membership, credentials offered, continuing education, student membership, and so on are listed. Make a comparison chart of both organizations discussing your findings. Explain which organization you want to join and which credential you hope to achieve and why.

APPLICATION ASSIGNMENT

You need to research the job market for your selected credential and or ideal job. Look at websites of employers where you wish to seek employment, local newspapers, professional organizational job banks, hiring websites (such as Monster or Indeed) and locate a job for which you want to apply. You will use this job to create a cover letter and resume to apply for it.

CRITICAL THINKING ASSIGNMENT

Reflect back on the AAPC and AHIMA professional organizations you researched. Research the local state component associations in your area. What are the local chapters or state organizations closest to you? Visit the website for those closest or the one you are most interested in joining, and review their website. Does the local or state association have annual, biannual, or quarterly meetings? If so, can students attend? Discuss what the benefit of attending one of these meetings would be for a student. Explain how a student can use this as a networking activity and why a professional network is important to have. Can a professional network benefit a student?

REVIEW QUESTIONS

1. Which of the following code sets is developed by the American Dental Association?
   a. CDT
   b. CPT
   c. HCPCS
   d. ICD-10-CM

2. _____ is the process of accurately assigning codes to verbal descriptions of patients' conditions and the healthcare services provided to treat those conditions.
   a. Abstracting
   b. Assigning
   c. Arranging
   d. Coding

3. When was HIPAA passed?
   a. 1983
   b. 1990
   c. 1996
   d. 2014

4. Before a coder can assign codes they _____ information from the medical record.
   a. abstract
   b. assign
   c. arrange
   d. code

5. The codes a coder _____ must accurately describe both the information documented in the medical record and the patient's condition and services.
   a. abstracts
   b. assigns
   c. arranges
   d. codes

6. When more than one diagnosis or procedure is required for the encounter, the coder must _____ the codes in a specific order.
   a. abstract
   b. assign
   c. arrange
   d. code

7. Which of the following is not an example of an outpatient encounter?
   a. ambulatory surgery
   b. cardiology lab
   c. intensive care unit
   d. physical therapy

8. Which of the following is used when a patient has been formally admitted to a healthcare facility?
   a. Inpatient encounter
   b. Outpatient encounter
   c. Observation encounter
   d. Transfer

9. Which of the following includes questions about current symptoms?
   a. History
   b. Physical exam
   c. Laboratory
   d. Diagnostic testing

10. How many steps are there in each encounter?
   a. 2
   b. 3
   c. 4
   d. 5

CODING AND REIMBURSEMENT

SCAVENGER HUNT

Go to the following website: http://www.cms.gov/Outreach-and-Education/
Medicare-Learning-Network-MLN/MLNProducts/downloads/MCRP_
Booklet.pdf and read the Medicare Claim Review Programs: MR, NCCI
Edits, MUEs, CERT and Recovery Audit Program. Write a one-page synopsis
of one of the five claim review programs discussing its role in the life cycle
of Medicare claims processing. Inside this booklet are web links, videos, and
other articles/newsletters to read. Click on one of these blue hyperlinked
articles or videos and discuss your findings. Explain how this knowledge will
help you as you enter the coding/reimbursement profession.

INTERVIEW WITH A CODER

Identify a coding or reimbursement professional, preferably a credentialed
one (RHIA, RHIT, CCS, CCS-P, CPC or CPC-H). Explain to this
professional that you are a student and have been given an assignment to
interview a coding/reimbursement professional.

Prepare 15 questions you would like to ask this coder, which may include the
following:

1. How did you first become interested in the coding/reimbursement
   profession?
2. How long have you been working in the coding/reimbursement
   profession and how did you get your start?
3. What professional certification do you have and how long have you
   held this credential?
4. How many health care settings have you worked in and do you have
   a favorite setting?
5. Is one setting harder to work in than the other? if so, why?
6. Which setting do you recommend a new student to start in?
7. What is one of the biggest challenges you have had to deal with on
   the job?
8. What is your favorite aspect of your job?
9. What is your least favorite aspect of your job?
10. What is the most rewarding part of your job?
11. What is the most aggravating part of your job?
12. What is a typical day like for you?

13. Do you need to go to continuing education every year? if so, how much?

14. Is there anything I can do as a student to get more prepared for the coding/reimbursement job market?

15. What is your advice for a new graduate trying to get a foot in the door.

Be sure to dress in business attire as if you were going to a job interview. Arrive to the facility/office 10 minutes early. At the conclusion of the interview, be sure to thank the professional for his/her time.

Write a paper listing the name and credentials of whom you interviewed, the place of his/her employment, the address for the employer, and the time and date of the interview. Include the questions you used as well as the answers. Include a reflection in the paper of how well you think you will like the daily work of this profession and if you feel it is the right profession for you.

Mail a handwritten thank you to the professional a few days after the interview to thank him/her again for their valuable time and help in your assignment completion.

CRITICAL THINKING ASSIGNMENT

Go to the CMS.gov website and watch a web-based training video on fraud and abuse.

Go to www.cms.gov/Outreach-and-Education/Medicare-Learning-Network-MLN/MLNEdWebGuide/Products_and_Resources_for_Billing_and_Coding.html

Under "Related Links", go to "Web-Based Training (WBT) Courses."

Click on "Avoiding Medicare Fraud and Abuse: A Roadmap for Physicians" (developed March 2012, revised November 2014).

https://cms.meridianksi.com/kc/main/pop_up_frm.asp?loc=/kc/ilc/course_info_enroll_info.asp%3Fpreview%3DFalse%26crs_ident%3DC00267&strFunction=width%3D200%2Cheight%3D100&strTable=undefined&strContentID=undefined

Watch the video and write a one-half to one-page summary of what you found most useful from this video and how this knowledge will help you as you enter the coding/reimbursement profession. Be sure to print off the CE credit certificate at the end and keep for your records.

REVIEW QUESTIONS

1. In which year was Medicare established?
   a. 1960
   b. 1965
   c. 1970
   d. 1975

2. Which part of Medicare covers physician services?
   a. Medicare Part A
   b. Medicare Part B
   c. Medicare Part C
   d. Medicare Part D

3. Which part of Medicare is also called Medicare Advantage?
   a. Medicare Part A
   b. Medicare Part B
   c. Medicare Part C
   d. Medicare Part D

4. Which of the following is a Medicare Supplemental insurance policy?
   a. Medicare Part D
   b. Medicaid
   c. Medigap
   d. Tricare

5. Which of the following was established in 1997?
   a. Tricare
   b. CHIP
   c. VHA
   d. WC

6. Which of the following pays for medical costs due to employment-related injuries?
   a. Tricare
   b. CHIP
   c. VHA
   d. WC

7. What percentage of Americans are covered by a group health plan?
   a. 40%
   b. 50%
   c. 60%
   d. 75%

8. Which of the following is not an example of medical necessity?
   a. Diagnosis: Hip dislocation treatment: physical therapy
   b. Diagnosis: lung cancer treatment: chemotherapy
   c. Diagnosis: astigmatism treatment: LASIX
   d. Diagnosis: Chronic tonsillitis treatment: tonsillectomy and adenoidectomy

9. Which of the following is true about excellent documentation?
   a. Can reduce the amount of time needed to code a claim
   b. Can result in more accurate coding
   c. Can result in more complete coding
   d. All of these are true

10. Which of the following would not be included in the PE?
    a. Neck: Supple
    b. Lungs: Wheezing heard throughout the lung fields
    c. Abdomen: Soft
    d. Labs: Fasting blood sugar is 130

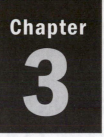
THE TRANSITION TO ICD-10

SCAVENGER HUNT

Go to www.medscape.org and read the article titled Transition to ICD-10: Getting Started www.medscape.org/viewarticle/765754

After reading the article write a one-page paper summarizing what you read and discuss why this article is important for coders to read. What was the biggest benefit to you as you read this article and why?

APPLICATION ASSIGNMENT

Using the ICD-9-CM Codes provided for the following scenarios go to www.icd10data.com and convert the following ICD-9 Codes into ICD-10-CM Codes.

1. Dehydration

   ICD-9-CM Diagnosis Code: 276.51

   ICD-10-CM Diagnosis Code:

2. Acute serous otitis media, left ear

   ICD-9-CM Diagnosis Code: 381.01

   ICD-10-CM Diagnosis Code:

3. Hypertension

   ICD-9-CM Diagnosis Code: 401.9

   ICD-10-CM Diagnosis Code:

4. UTI

   ICD-9-CM Diagnosis Code: 599.0

   ICD-10-CM Diagnosis Code:

5. Pneumonia

   ICD-9-CM Diagnosis Code: 486

   ICD-10-CM Diagnosis Code:

6. COPD

   ICD-9-CM Diagnosis Code: 496

   ICD-10-CM Diagnosis Code:

7. Anemia

   ICD-9-CM Diagnosis Code: 285.9

   ICD-10-CM Diagnosis Code:

8. Hypertrophy of tonsils and adenoids

   ICD-9-CM Diagnosis Code: 474.10

   ICD-10-CM Diagnosis Code:

9. Mild intellectual disabilities

   ICD-9-CM Diagnosis Code: 317

   ICD-10-CM Diagnosis Code:

10. Low back pain

    ICD-9-CM Diagnosis Code: 724.2

    ICD-10-CM Diagnosis Code:

CRITICAL THINKING ASSIGNMENT

Go to www.cms.gov and pull up the 2015 General Equivalence Mappings (GEMS) – Diagnosis Codes and Guide www.cms.gov/Medicare/Coding/ICD10/2015-ICD-10-CM-and-GEMs.html

After you read this document write a one-page paper discussing the purpose of the GEMs and how you think you might use this resource as a coder.

REVIEW QUESTIONS

1. What does ICD-10 stand for?
   a. International Classification of Diseases, 10th Revision
   b. International Classification of Diseases, 10th Year
   c. International Categories of Diseases, 10th Revision
   d. International Categories of Diseases, 10th Year

2. Who developed ICD-10-PCS?
   a. AMA
   b. AHA
   c. CMS
   d. WHO

3. Who developed ICD-10?
   a. AMA
   b. AHA
   c. CMS
   d. WHO

4. How many codes are in the ICD-10-PCS system?
   a. 3,000
   b. 16,000
   c. 70,000
   d. 72,000

5. Which of the following is not a benefit of ICD-10-CM?
   a. Codes describe patient conditions more accurately.
   b. Codes provide more detail.
   c. Code provide higher quality data.
   d. All of these are benefits.

6. How many characters are in an ICD-10-CM Code?
   a. 3 digits
   b. 5 digits
   c. 7 digits
   d. Up to 7 digits

7. How many characters are in an ICD-10-PCS Code?
   a. 3 digits
   b. 5 digits
   c. 7 digits
   d. Up to 7 digits

8. What are some documentation changes physicians are going to have to make to prepare for the new ICD-10 Coding system?
   a. Include laterality
   b. Include anatomic specificity
   c. None of these
   d. All of these

9. Which of the following will be required for coders to increase their knowledge of before the new ICD-10 Coding system?
   a. Anatomy and Physiology
   b. Medical Terminology
   c. Pathophysiology
   d. All of these

10. In ICD-10-CM how many codes are there for falls?
    a. 20
    b. 40
    c. 100
    d. 300

SCAVENGER HUNT

Go to AHIMA and search for the following document: "Frequently asked questions about ICD-10-CM/PCS" or just go to the following link:

http://library.ahima.org/xpedio/groups/public/documents/ahima/bok1_050729.pdf

Read all the questions and answers located on this document and report on three of these. Why did you have the same question and what did you learn from the answer AHIMA provided?

APPLICATION ASSIGNMENT

Abstracting Medical Documentation

Read the following discharge summary and abstract out information needed to code this chart.

ADMITTING DIAGNOSIS: Abscess with cellulitis, left foot.

DISCHARGE DIAGNOSIS: Status post I&D, left foot.

PROCEDURES: Incision and drainage, first metatarsal head, left foot with culture and sensitivity.

HISTORY OF PRESENT ILLNESS: The patient presented to Dr. X's office on 06/14/07 complaining of a painful left foot. The patient had been treated conservatively in office for approximately 5 days, but symptoms progressed with the need of incision and drainage being decided.

MEDICATIONS: Ancef IV.

ALLERGIES: ACCUTANE.

SOCIAL HISTORY: Denies smoking or drinking.

PHYSICAL EXAMINATION: Palpable pedal pulses noted bilaterally. Capillary refill time less than 3 seconds, digits 1 through 5 bilateral.

Skin supple and intact with positive hair growth. Epicritic sensation intact bilateral. Muscle strength +5/5, dorsiflexors, plantar flexors, invertors, evertors. Left foot with erythema, edema, positive tenderness noted, left forefoot area.

LABORATORY: White blood cell count never was abnormal. The remaining within normal limits. X-ray is negative for osteomyelitis. On 06/14/07, the patient was taken to the OR for incision and drainage of left foot abscess. The patient tolerated the procedure well and was admitted and placed on vancomycin 1 g q.12h after surgery and later changed Ancef 2 g IV every 8 hours. Postop wound care consists of Aquacel Ag and dry dressing to the surgical site every day and the patient remains nonweightbearing on the left foot. The patient progressively improved with IV antibiotics and local wound care and was discharged from the hospital on 06/19/07 in excellent condition.

DISCHARGE MEDICATIONS: Lorcet 10/650 mg, dispense 24 tablets, one tablet to be taken by mouth q.6h as needed for pain. The patient was continued on Ancef 2 g IV via PICC line and home health administration of IV antibiotics.

DISCHARGE INSTRUCTIONS: Included keeping the foot elevated with long periods of rest. The patient is to wear surgical shoe at all times for ambulation and to avoid excessive ambulation. The patient to keep dressing dry and intact, left foot. The patient to contact Dr. X for all follow-up care, if any problems arise. The patient was given written and oral instruction about wound care before discharge. Prior to discharge, the patient was noted to be afebrile. All vitals were stable. The patient's questions were answered and the patient was discharged in apparent satisfactory condition. Follow-up care was given via Dr. X's office.

Report taken from MTsamples.com (http://mtsamples.com/site/pages/sample.asp?Type=89-Discharge%20Summary&Sample=1254-Abscess%20with%20Cellulitis%20-%20Discharge%20Summary)

Table 4-7 in your text lists out some key criteria for abstracting diagnoses. See which of the following information is contained in this discharge summary:

1. What is the gender and age of patient?

2. What is the patient's chief complaint or reason for admission?

3. Was the patient an inpatient or outpatient?

4. What symptoms and signs are described?

5. Does the physician provide a definitive diagnosis?

6. Does the physician provided a diagnosis that is uncertain, probable, possible, qualified, or rule out?

7. Which symptoms and signs are integral to the definitive diagnosis?

8. Which symptoms and signs are related, but not integral, to the definitive diagnosis?

9. What unrelated conditions, symptoms, or signs are managed during the encounter?

10. What conditions, symptoms, or signs are not managed during the encounter?

11. What is the laterality, if any, of the condition?

12. What is the treatment plan or procedure? Is it consistent with the diagnosis?

13. Is the condition the result of an injury or external cause?

CRITICAL THINKING ASSIGNMENT

For the discharge summary that you just abstracted, what ICD-10-CM Diagnosis Code(s) would you assign:

ICD-10-CM Diagnosis Code(s):

CODING CASES

Instructions: For each of the diagnostic statements, look up the main term in your alphabetic index, verify the code in the tabular list, and assign the correct ICD-10-CM Diagnosis Code.

1. Blepharitis of the left lower eyelid: ICD-10-CM Code _____

2. Corbus' disease: ICD-10-CM Code _____

3. Delhi boil: ICD-10-CM Code _____

4. Patient came to the emergency room with complaints of orthopnea: ICD-10-CM Code _____

5. Plaque psoriasis: ICD-10-CM Code _____

6. Fluid overload: ICD-10-CM Code _____

7. Cluster headache: ICD-10-CM Code _____

8. Chronic mucoid otitis media, bilateral: ICD-10-CM Code _____

9. Terminal atrophy of kidney: ICD-10-CM Code _____

10. Acute follicular conjunctivitis, right eye: ICD-10-CM Code _____

NEOPLASMS

SCAVENGER HUNT

Read the following article on Neoplasm Coding in ICD-10 versus ICD-9. http://www.justcoding.com/283813/specificity-key-to-neoplasm-coding-in-icd10cm.

Discuss how this article will benefit you as you start neoplasm coding and why coders need to understand that difference in neoplasm coding guidelines between ICD-9 and ICD-10. Which one element of this article did you find the most beneficial, and why?

APPLICATION ASSIGNMENT

Matching Neoplasm Terms:

_____ 1. Direct extension
_____ 2. Invasive
_____ 3. Metastasis
_____ 4. Neoplasm
_____ 5. Benign
_____ 6. Ca in situ
_____ 7. Uncertain behavior
_____ 8. Unspecified behavior

a. a noninvasive neoplasm that does not spread to other sites
b. the invasion of adjacent sites by a malignant neoplasm
c. malignant tumor cells that are confined to the point of origin
d. the extension of tumor cells to other adjacent sites
e. the behavior of the neoplasm cannot be determined at the time it was discovered
f. the resulting spread of invasive tumor cells
g. neither the behavior of the tumor nor the morphology of the tumor is identified
h. a new or abnormal growth

CRITICAL THINKING ASSIGNMENT

Select one of the Official Guidelines for Coding and Reporting that deals with neoplasms from those in Section I. C.2 a-r (the official guidelines can be found at http://www.cdc.gov/nchs/data/icd/ICD10cmguidelines_2015%209_26_2014.pdf).

Describe what the guideline is saying and how we will use this in coding. Give a scenario example of when this guideline would be applied.

CODING CASES

1. Carcinoma of the tail of the pancreas: ICD-10-CM Diagnosis Code _____

2. Neoplasm of the breast: ICD-10-CM Diagnosis Code _____

3. Adenocarcinoma of the right cornea: ICD-10-CM Diagnosis Code _____

4. Carcinoma of the medulla of the left adrenal gland: ICD-10-CM Diagnosis Code _____

5. Metastatic carcinoma of the left kidney and renal pelvis: ICD-10-CM Diagnosis Code _____

6. Hepatic cell carcinoma: ICD-10-CM Diagnosis Code _____

7. Adenoma of the skin of the majora labia: ICD-10-CM Diagnosis Code _____

8. Adenocarcinoma of the cecum: ICD-10-CM Diagnosis Code _____

9. Melanoma of the external skin of the right ear: ICD-10-CM Diagnosis Code _____

10. Lipoma of the kidney: ICD-10-CM Diagnosis Code _____

11. Carcinoma in situ of the bladder: ICD-10-CM Diagnosis Code _____

12. Metastatic melanoma from the left lateral chest wall to the axillary lymph node: ICD-10-CM Diagnosis Codes _____

13. Gliosarcoma: ICD-10-CM Diagnosis Code _____

14. Dermoid of the right ovary: ICD-10-CM Diagnosis Code _____

15. B-cell lymphoma of the intra-abdominal lymph nodes: ICD-10-CM Diagnosis Code _____

16. Patient with multiple myeloma who is currently in relapse: ICD-10-CM Diagnosis Code _____

17. Hemangioma of the liver: ICD-10-CM Diagnosis Code _____

18. Blastoma of the left lower lobe of the lung: ICD-10-CM Diagnosis Code _____

19. Patient with acute myelomonocytic leukemia who is currently in remission: ICD-10-CM Diagnosis Code _____

20. Carcinoma of the right upper lobe of the bronchus with metastasis to the intrathoracic lymph nodes: ICD-10-CM Diagnosis Codes _____

CODING PRACTICE CASES

Case 1

Read the following coding scenario, and apply the applicable ICD-10-CM Diagnosis Code(s):

Ms. Jane Dotty is a pleasant 46-year-old Caucasian female who first palpated a mass in the left breast last fall. The mass increased in size since her initial visit last fall. The patient underwent biopsy of the mass, which shows stage II breast cancer of the lower-outer quadrant of the left breast. Patient is being scheduled for a radical mastectomy of the left breast and will be evaluated by Dr. Francesca for chemotherapy after surgery. What is the correct ICD-10-CM Diagnosis Code(s) assigned?

Case 2

Read the following coding scenario and apply the applicable ICD-10-CM diagnosis code(s):

Mr. Cooper Conrad is a young man who was referred to me by his dentist. Mr. Conrad is a 28-year-old Hispanic male who was found to have buccal leukoplakia during his routine dental cleaning two weeks ago. A biopsy of his buccal mucosa was completed and the pathology report revealed carcinoma in situ of the buccal mucosa. What is the correct ICD-10-CM Diagnosis Code(s) assigned?

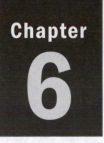

SYMPTOMS, SIGNS, ABNORMAL CLINICAL AND LABORATORY FINDINGS

SCAVENGER HUNT

Go to HCPRO and read the following article:

http://blogs.hcpro.com/icd-10/2013/07/signs-symptoms-and-unspecified-codes/

Then think about how signs/symptoms play a role in a physician's documentation and how you, the coder, need to interpret the documentation and decide what signs/symptoms are integral to a diagnosis/disease/condition documented by the physician. Then go to the Merck Manual, www .merckmanual.com/home, and click on Consumer version. In the top right is a search magnifying glass, click on this and enter a disease that you want to research (i.e., Pneumonia).

Hit the medical topic that you want to review after you entered your search term, and read about the medical topic. Discuss what the signs/symptoms are of this topic and how this knowledge is important for us to understand in coding. Provide a scenario in which a patient has a condition, with or without symptoms, and discuss how this would be coded. List out the codes you would assign and the rationale for these codes.

APPLICATION ASSIGNMENT

Go to a pharmaceutical reference, such as www.drugs.com, and research 20 signs/symptoms and the medicines most frequently used to treat each of them. Discuss why, as a coder, it is important to understand medicines and their relationship to diagnoses.

CRITICAL THINKING ASSIGNMENT

Select one of the Official Coding Guidelines that deals with Sign/Symptom Coding from those in Section I. B.4, B.18, C.18 a–h or Section II. A. (the official guidelines can be found at http://www.cdc.gov/nchs/data/icd/icd10cm_guidelines_2014.pdf).

Describe what the guideline is saying and how we will use this in coding. Give a scenario example of when this guideline would be applied.

CODING CASES

1. Rapid heartbeat: ICD-10-CM Diagnosis Code_____

2. Hyperglycemia: ICD-10-CM Diagnosis Code_____

3. Slurred speech: ICD-10-CM Diagnosis Code_____

4. Pins and needles sensation of the skin: ICD-10-CM Diagnosis Code_____

5. Cardiogenic shock: ICD-10-CM Diagnosis Code_____

6. Patient with a lack of energy: ICD-10-CM Diagnosis Code_____

7. Infant who is a fussy baby: ICD-10-CM Diagnosis Code_____

8. Patient with an abnormal blood level of zinc: ICD-10-CM Diagnosis Code_____

9. Patient who had a mammogram that showed dense breasts: ICD-10-CM Diagnosis Code_____

10. Excessive thirst: ICD-10-CM Diagnosis Code_____

11. Patient with severe halitosis: ICD-10-CM Diagnosis Code_____

12. Fluid retention: ICD-10-CM Diagnosis Code_____

13. Patient with absent bowel sounds during examination: ICD-10-CM Diagnosis Code_____

14. Loss of voice: ICD-10-CM Diagnosis Code_____

15. Albuminuria: ICD-10-CM Diagnosis Code_____

16. Headache: ICD-10-CM Diagnosis Code_____

17. Patient with an unexplained facial droop: ICD-10-CM Diagnosis Code_____

18. Petechiae: ICD-10-CM Diagnosis Code_____

19. Patient being seen for 2 days of nausea and vomiting: ICD-10-CM Diagnosis Code_____

20. Nosebleed: ICD-10-CM Diagnosis Code_____

CODING PRACTICE CASES

Case 1

Joey Jelly is seen in the ER today for fainting. The triage nurse takes his vitals, which reveal a temperature of 99°F, blood pressure at 118/70, and weight at 195. The physician completes an examination of the patient without any abnormal findings. A blood panel is ordered to evaluate the patient's chemistry. The blood tests all return normal, and the physician documents near-syncope episode. What is the correct ICD-10-CM Diagnosis Code(s) assigned?

Case 2

Hannah Holiday is brought to the office today by her mother. Hannah is 18 months old, and her parents are very concerned that she is not walking yet. Hannah does sit up and will roll to get items she desires but never crawled or walked. Her mother indicates that she is the first baby, and they do have a habit of holding her a lot. The physician completes an exam and reviews her reflexes. He does not find any abnormalities. The physician would like the mother to take Hannah to a physical therapist for gait training. What is the correct ICD-10-CM Diagnosis Code(s) assigned?

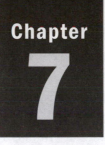
FACTORS INFLUENCING HEALTH STATUS AND CONTACT WITH HEALTH SERVICES

SCAVENGER HUNT

Read the following article from AHIMA: http://library.ahima.org/xpedio/groups/public/documents/ahima/bok1_049298.hcsp?dDocName= bok1_049298

Discuss the importance of Z codes and why you think that Z codes accounted for 20% of all outpatient visits. Browse through the Z code tabular index and select five diagnosis codes that you think are commonly used for outpatient visits, and discuss why.

APPLICATION ASSIGNMENT

There are certain Z codes that may only be the principal diagnosis. List what these codes are, and discuss the importance of recognizing these as a coder. What can happen if one of the principal diagnosis-only Z codes is not listed as the principal diagnosis?

CRITICAL THINKING ASSIGNMENT

Select one of the Official Coding Guidelines that deals with Factors Influencing Health Status Coding from those in Section I. C.21 a–c (the official guidelines can be found at http://www.cdc.gov/nchs/data/icd/ICD10cmguidelines_2015%209_26_2014.pdf).

Describe what the guideline is saying and how we will use this in coding. Give a scenario example of when this guideline would be applied.

CODING CASES

1. Healthy newborn baby check for a newborn 12 days old: ICD-10-CM Diagnosis Code_____

2. Patient who is being seen for bereavement of a family member: ICD-10-CM Diagnosis Code_____

3. Encounter for screening for prostate cancer: ICD-10-CM Diagnosis Code_____

4. A 23-year-old patient being seen for fertility testing: ICD-10-CM Diagnosis Code_____

5. Patient being seen today for dietary counseling. The physician is concerned about the patient's tobacco use, lack of physical exercise, and inappropriate dietary intake: ICD-10-CM Diagnosis Code(s)_____

6. Patient being seen for a breast lump who has a personal history of breast cancer 5 years ago: ICD-10-CM Diagnosis Code_____

7. The patient is an 11-year-old female being seen for mental health services after being abused by her biological father. The father has been removed from the home: ICD-10-CM Diagnosis Code_____

8. Allergy to penicillin: ICD-10-CM Diagnosis Code_____

9. Patient coming in today as she was exposed to anthrax and is now concerned about her health: ICD-10-CM Diagnosis Code_____

10. Patient who is status post-amputation of his right arm, above his elbow: ICD-10-CM Diagnosis Code_____

11. Patient being transferred to an SNF for dependence on a respirator so he is unable to go home at this time: ICD-10-CM Diagnosis Code_____

12. Homeless man presents to the ER to see if help can be given to him as he has nowhere to go: ICD-10-CM Diagnosis Code_____

13. Status post-automatic cardiac defibrillator: ICD-10-CM Diagnosis Code_____

14. A 24-year-old patient with muscular dystrophy who is confined to a wheelchair: ICD-10-CM Diagnosis Code(s)_____

15. Mom brought 7-year-old in to be seen today, as she is worried about his school performance. He has failed all school examinations, and she would like an evaluation. ICD-10-CM Diagnosis Code_____

16. A 23-year-old being seen in the office today for an IUD insertion: ICD-10-CM Diagnosis Code_____

17. An 88-year-old male seen today for atypical chest pain. He takes aspirin daily and has done so for 5 years: ICD-10-CM Diagnosis Code(s)_____

18. A 16-year-old comes to the clinic today scared that she is pregnant. A pregnancy test was completed, which confirmed that she is pregnant. The patient was referred to Planned Parenthood to discuss her situation with counselors there: ICD-10-CM Diagnosis Code_____

19. Mary Jane, a 19-year-old, is brought to the ER by two friends. They were all at a party this evening when Mary Jane was raped by a fellow college student. The physician completed a rape examination and testing kit, and police were notified: ICD-10-CM Diagnosis Code_____

20. Al Allup, a 60-year-old male, is seen today for a severe headache. Al complains that this has been going on for 3 days, and he is very scared, as his father died from a stroke at age 60: ICD-10-CM Diagnosis Code(s)_____

CODING PRACTICE CASES

Case 1

John Jordan, a 36-year-old male, was brought to the SDS suite this morning for a hernia repair. John has an indirect left inguinal hernia. The nurse checks John in, and during his questioning it was discovered that he ate breakfast this morning and now cannot have the surgery. The nurse explained that this is a contraindication for receiving anesthesia and that the procedure must be completed without any food or drink after midnight. The procedure is not completed and will be rescheduled for another day. Patient is sent home with instructions to call to office tomorrow to reschedule the surgery. ICD-10-CM Diagnosis Code(s)_____

Case 2

Mary Molls is a 55-year-old being seen today for chemotherapy administration. Today will be her second of five round of chemotherapy to treat her colon cancer. Mary has Stage II adenocarcinoma of the ascending colon. She responded well to the first round of chemotherapy. She received the chemotherapy without any complications and will return in 1 week for the third round of her chemotherapy. ICD-10-CM Diagnosis Code(s)_____

EXTERNAL CAUSES
OF MORBIDITY

SCAVENGER HUNT

Go to www.justcoding.com and read the following article:

http://www.justcoding.com/286867/complete-the-patients-story-with
-icd10cm-external-cause-codes

Discuss the importance of external cause codes and how you feel about the
mandatory use of these. Do you feel there should be mandatory reporting
of all external cause codes by all providers and facilities? Why or why not?
What are some benefits we get from having external cause codes? If we stop
and think about the quality of statistics, can external cause codes play a role
in that? Why or why not?

APPLICATION ASSIGNMENT

According to the Official ICD-10-CM Coding Guidelines, there are
sequencing rules to follow if two or more separate events cause separate
injuries (ICD-10-CM Coding Guideline 20.C.f). What is the order we follow
for listing which external cause code is first?

CRITICAL THINKING ASSIGNMENT

Select one of the Official Coding Guidelines that deals with External
Cause Coding from those in Section I. C.20 a-e or g-k (the offi-
cial guidelines can be found at http://www.cdc.gov/nchs/data/icd/
ICD10cmguidelines_2015%209_26_2014.pdf).

Describe what the guideline is saying and how we will use this in coding.
Give a scenario example of when this guideline would be applied.

CODING CASES

1. A 7-year-old who fell off his skateboard today: ICD-10-CM Diagnosis Code_____

2. Patient who drowned after their sailboat overturned: ICD-10-CM Diagnosis Code_____

3. Place of occurrence was the bathroom in a prison: ICD-10-CM Diagnosis Code_____

4. Chris was at the football arena when he was struck by a football during his football team's practice today after school: ICD-10-CM Diagnosis Code(s)_____

5. Patient was swimming today when she was struck by a ski boat: ICD-10-CM Diagnosis Code_____

6. Volunteer activity: ICD-10-CM Diagnosis Code_____

7. Activity is cross-country skiing: ICD-10-CM Diagnosis Code_____

8. Kicked by a cow while milking it: ICD-10-CM Diagnosis Code(s)_____

9. John tripped while playing ultimate Frisbee at the city park earlier today: ICD-10-CM Diagnosis Code(s)_____

10. Accidental handgun discharge: ICD-10-CM Diagnosis Code_____

11. Today Sally was seen for a blood transfusion. She was in hospital room 342A and was given excessive amounts of blood during her blood transfusion at the city hospital: ICD-10-CM Diagnosis Code(s)_____

12. Halley was enjoying a hot air balloon ride today until it crashed, injuring her and the other passengers: ICD-10-CM Diagnosis Code_____

13. Earthquake: ICD-10-CM Diagnosis Code_____

14. Place of occurrence was the swimming pool at the patient's family home: ICD-10-CM Diagnosis Code_____

15. Activity was vacuuming: ICD-10-CM Diagnosis Code_____

16. Patient fell today while ice skating at the city's outdoor skating arena: ICD-10-CM Diagnosis Code(s)_____

17. Patient was bitten about an hour ago by her pet macaw: ICD-10-CM Diagnosis Code_____

18. Cut with a knife: ICD-10-CM Diagnosis Code_____

19. Patient fell down the steps of his single-family home today walking out to get the mail. The steps were covered with ice: ICD-10-CM Diagnosis Code(s)_____

20. A 5-year-old knocked over by dog as she took him for a walk: ICD-10-CM Diagnosis Code(s)_____

CODING PRACTICE CASES

Case 1

Brad Bentely is a school bus driver. He was driving his school bus when a deer ran in front of him today on the way back to the bus garage after his school route. His bus hit the deer. He complains of neck pain and is taken to the ER. The ER physician examines the patient and determines he is suffering from whiplash. Whiplash instructions are given to the patient, and he is discharged home to return if his symptoms worsen: ICD-10-CM Diagnosis Code(s)_____

Case 2

Carly Jo was working in the kitchen at Shady Acres Nursing home when she broke a glass and cut her finger. The DNS evaluated Carly for a laceration to her right index finger. The DNS placed some Steri-Strips on Carly's finger and indicated that she did not believe sutures were necessary. Carly returned back to work on light duty for the rest of the night. ICD-10-CM Diagnosis Code(s)_____

DISEASES OF
THE DIGESTIVE SYSTEM

SCAVENGER HUNT

Go to www.hcpro.com, and read the following blog: http://blogs.hcpro.com/icd-10/2013/03/gerd-yourself-for-coding-digestive-diseases-in-icd-10-cm/

The blog discusses that when we are coding digestive system ulcers, we need to know the location as well as whether it was acute or chronic with hemorrhage or perforation or without hemorrhage or perforation. Discuss the locations of these ulcers: gastric, duodenal, peptic, and gastrojejunal. Then discuss what the difference is between acute and chronic and how we will know if an ulcer has hemorrhage and/or perforation. What would you look for in the documentation to decide which code to select when coding a digestive system ulcer?

APPLICATION ASSIGNMENT

Label the following diagram.

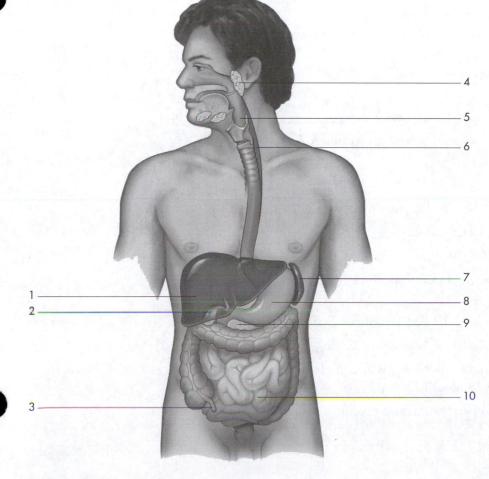

CRITICAL THINKING ASSIGNMENT

Select one of the Official Coding Guidelines that deals with Digestive Coding from those in Section I. C.2 11 (the official guidelines can be found at http://www.cdc.gov/nchs/data/icd/ICD10cmguidelines_2015%209_26_2014.pdf).

Section 11 does not contain anything and is reserved for future guideline expansion, so look at the Section II Guidelines, A–K, and select one of these to discuss.

Describe what the guideline is saying and how we will use this in coding. Give a scenario example of when this guideline would be applied.

CODING CASES

1. Acute appendicitis with generalized peritonitis: ICD-10-CM Diagnosis Code_____

2. Sialolithiasis: ICD-10-CM Diagnosis Code_____

3. John is being seen today for Barrett's esophagus with low-grade dysplasia: ICD-10-CM Diagnosis Code_____

4. Hillary Hill is being seen today for evaluation of her Crohn's disease: ICD-10-CM Diagnosis Code_____

5. Strangulation of the small intestine: ICD-10-CM Diagnosis Code_____

6. Cholelithiasis with chronic cholecystitis: ICD-10-CM Diagnosis Code_____

7. Whipple's disease: ICD-10-CM Diagnosis Code_____

8. Patient is seen today for left-sided colitis with fistula: ICD-10-CM Diagnosis Code_____

9. Hepatic angiomatosis: ICD-10-CM Diagnosis Code_____

10. Ulcerative stomatitis: ICD-10-CM Diagnosis Code_____

11. Hematemsis: ICD-10-CM Diagnosis Code_____

12. Stomatitis herpetiformis: ICD-10-CM Diagnosis Code_____

13. Acute gastrojejunal ulcer with perforation: ICD-10-CM Diagnosis Code_____

14. Stenosis of the duodenum: ICD-10-CM Diagnosis Code_____

15. Pseudocyst of pancreas: ICD-10-CM Diagnosis Code_____

16. Patient was discovered to have colon polyps and grade III anal hemorrhoids: ICD-10-CM Diagnosis Code(s)_____

17. Diverticulitis of colon with perforation and bleeding: ICD-10-CM Diagnosis Code_____

18. Kathy is been seen today for maintenance of her gluten-sensitive enteropathy: ICD-10-CM Diagnosis Code_____

19. Toxic liver disease with chronic active hepatitis: ICD-10-CM Diagnosis Code_____

20. Recurrent right-sided femoral hernia with obstruction: ICD-10-CM Diagnosis Code_____

CODING PRACTICE CASES

Case 1

William Williamson is a 45-year-old Caucasian male brought into the ER for severe abdominal pain. The patient is unable to stand up straight as the pain is very severe. Mr. Williamson smells of alcohol and admits to the nurse that he drank before he arrived at the ER. The ER physician calls Dr. Smith, an internist, who admits Mr. Williamson to his care. Dr. Smith orders some labs and an abdominal ultrasound. Upon review of the patient's history it is discovered that he is a heavy drinker. He admits to drinking one bottle of hard alcohol, typically vodka, per night. After the lab and radiology results are in, Dr. Smith determines that the patient has alcoholic gastritis with bleeding due to alcohol dependence with current intoxication: ICD-10-CM Diagnosis Code(s)_____

Case 2

Ava Avalon is a 5-year-old Hispanic female brought to the ER today by her mother for nausea and vomiting. The mother reports that they ate dinner about 2 hours ago and then Ava started vomiting profusely and has not stopped. The mother is getting worried as Ava is typically very healthy. The physician completes a history and physical and performs an examination. The physician is concerned that she might have food poisoning and asks the mother what they had for dinner. The mother stated that they had shellfish, and Ava really liked these, as it was her first time. The physician orders some lab work and determines that Ava is suffering from an allergic gastroenteritis due to shellfish. He explains to the mother that Ava is allergic to shellfish and that she should follow up with her family physician for further allergy testing: ICD-10-CM Diagnosis Code_____

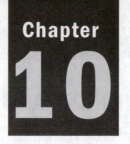

ENDOCRINE, NUTRITIONAL, AND METABOLIC DISEASES

SCAVENGER HUNT

Go to www.ahima.org and read the following article: http://journal.ahima .org/2012/05/16/coding-diabetes-mellitus-in-icd-10-cm-4/

Discuss why we need to understand the intricacies of coding diabetic conditions. Discuss a few complications we might see when coding diabetes, and include the code(s) associated to code for diabetes plus the complication. Look at the last scenario in this article: Coding for Diabetes Mellitus with Insulin Pump. Then look at the question at the bottom posted from a reader.

"I came across this article online and thought is full of great information, however, I have a question relating to the example for coding DM with insulin pump. The dx was type I DM with leaking insulin pump. I do not think code E08.69 is correct to capture the type 1 DM. It is my understanding that E08 is used for secondary DM, not type I. There may have been a correction in subsequent journals, but I did not locate it. Can someone confirm if E08.69 is correct? Thank you. Respectfully, Valerie."

What do you think the correct answer is for her question? Be sure to support your answer.

APPLICATION ASSIGNMENT

Match the following hormones to the correct endocrine gland:

_____ 1. Pituitary gland
_____ 2. Pineal gland
_____ 3. Thyroid gland
_____ 4. Parathyroid gland
_____ 5. Pancreas
_____ 6. Adrenal cortex gland
_____ 7. Adrenal medulla gland
_____ 8. Ovaries
_____ 9. Testes
_____ 10. Thymus gland

a. Melantonin, serotonin
b. Glucagon, insulin, somatostatin
c. Cortisol, aldosterone, testosterone, androsterone
d. testosterone
e. Dopamine, Epinephrine (adrenaline), norepinephrine (noradrenaline)
f. Thyroxine, triiodothyronine, calcitonin
g. Estrogens, progesterone
h. Growth hormone, follicle-stimulating hormone, prolactin hormone, oxytocin, antidiuretic hormone
i. Thymosin, thymopoietin
j. Parathyroid hormone

CRITICAL THINKING ASSIGNMENT

Select one of the Official Coding Guidelines that deals with Endocrine Coding from those in Section I. C.4 a (the official guidelines can be found at http://www.cdc.gov/nchs/data/icd/ICD10cmguidelines_2015%209_26_2014 .pdf).

Describe what the guideline is saying and how we will use this in coding. Give a scenario example of when this guideline would be applied.

CODING CASES

1. Type I diabetes mellitus with mild nonproliferative diabetic retinopathy with macular edema: ICD-10-CM Diagnosis Code_____

2. Bartter's syndrome: ICD-10-CM Diagnosis Code_____

3. A 6-year-old being seen today for night blindness. It is determined that her night blindness is due to a vitamin A deficiency: ICD-10-CM Diagnosis Code_____

4. Billy is being seen today for hypersecretion of testicular hormones: ICD-10-CM Diagnosis Code_____

5. Vitamin E deficiency: ICD-10-CM Diagnosis Code_____

6. A 1-year-old is being followed up today at the office for her congenital lactase deficiency: ICD-10-CM Diagnosis Code_____

7. A 17-year-old who has been sick for a week and is being treated today for dehydration: ICD-10-CM Diagnosis Code_____

8. Addison's disease: ICD-10-CM Diagnosis Code_____

9. Myoclonic epilepsy without status epilepticus with associated ragged-red fibers (MERRF syndrome): ICD-10-CM Diagnosis Code(s)_____

10. Type I diabetes mellitus with diabetic amyotrophy: ICD-10-CM Diagnosis Code_____

11. HGPRT deficiency: ICD-10-CM Diagnosis Code_____

12. Adrenomyeloneuropathy: ICD-10-CM Diagnosis Code_____

13. Hypertrophy of the thymus: ICD-10-CM Diagnosis Code_____

14. A 77-year-old admitted to ICU today in respiratory alkalosis: ICD-10-CM Diagnosis Code_____

15. Type D Niemann-Pick disease: ICD-10-CM Diagnosis Code_____

16. Zollinger-Ellison syndrome: ICD-10-CM Diagnosis Code_____

17. Patient is being seen today to discuss his morbid obesity. It is determined that his morbid obesity is due to an excessive amount of caloric intake daily, and it is recommended that he meet with a dietician to get on a weight-loss plan: ICD-10-CM Diagnosis Code_____

18. Tay-Sachs disease: ICD-10-CM Diagnosis Code_____

19. A 7-year-old patient seen today for juvenile osteomalacia: ICD-10-CM Diagnosis Code_____

20. Type 2 DM with diabetic polyneuropathy: ICD-10-CM Diagnosis Code_____

CODING PRACTICE CASES

Case 1

Lilly Little is transferred to the hospital today from the nursing home she is a resident at for a chronic foot ulcer that they cannot seem to get under control. Dr. Jones admits Ms. Little to the medical floor and evaluates her ulcer. Upon evaluation Dr. Jones determines that her ulcer is a nonpressure ulcer that is associated with necrosis of the muscle. He orders PT to complete debridement and whirlpool therapy to remove any necrotic skin and promote healing. Dr. Jones's final diagnosis is Type I diabetes with foot ulcer: ICD-10-CM Diagnosis Code(s)_____

Case 2

Kale Krew is seen in the ER today for fatigue, muscle weakness, and a headache. He complains that his whole body hurts and it has for about 2 weeks, to the point that he is unable to concentrate at work. The ER physician consults with Dr. James, in general medicine, and Mr. Krew was admitted for workup and screening. Dr. James orders a CB, and other lab panels to evaluate Mr. Krew's hormone level. After workup is complete, it is determined that Mr. Krew has Cushing syndrome and obesity. Dr. James prescribes Nizoral and advises Mr. Krew to meet with a dietician to determine an effective weight-loss strategy. ICD-10-CM Diagnosis Code(s)_____

DISEASES OF THE SKIN AND SUBCUTANEOUS TISSUE

SCAVENGER HUNT

Go to the website ICD10monitor and read the following article:
http://www.icd10monitor.com/asc/317-skin-ulcer-coding-in-icd-10-cm?showall=&limitstart=

Included in the article are sample exercises, and the answers are supplied at the end. Complete all the sample exercises, and discuss the codes you assigned for each exercise. Supply the rationale for each assigned code. Then compare the answers supplied at the end. How did you do? What did you learn from reading the article, completing the exercises, and comparing the correct answers?

APPLICATION ASSIGNMENT

Anatomy Labeling. Please identify the structures of the integumentary system in the following figure by filling in the blanks.

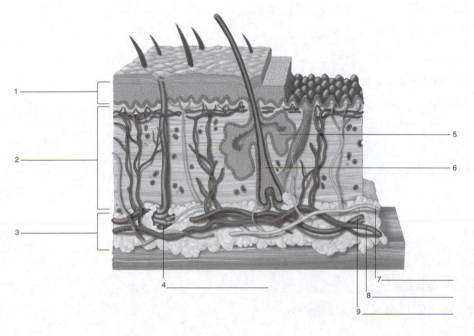

CRITICAL THINKING

Select one of the Official Coding Guidelines that deals with Diseases of Skin and Subcutaneous Tissue Coding from those in Section I. C.12 a (the official guidelines can be found at http://www.cdc.gov/nchs/data/icd/ICD10cmguidelines_2015%209_26_2014.pdf).

Describe what the guideline is saying and how we will use this in coding. Give a scenario example of when this guideline would be applied.

CODING CASES

1. Plaque psoriasis: ICD-10-CM Diagnosis Code_____

2. Allergic dermatitis due to dog dander: ICD-10-CM Diagnosis Code_____

3. Premature graying of the hair: ICD-10-CM Diagnosis Code_____

4. Pressure ulcer, stage 1, left elbow: ICD-10-CM Diagnosis Code_____

5. Striae atrophicae: ICD-10-CM Diagnosis Code_____

6. Boil of right axilla: ICD-10-CM Diagnosis Code_____

7. Erythema intertrigo: ICD-10-CM Diagnosis Code_____

8. Dry skin dermatitis: ICD-10-CM Diagnosis Code_____

9. Fibrosis of skin: ICD-10-CM Diagnosis Code_____

10. Lichen myxedematosus: ICD-10-CM Diagnosis Code_____

11. Pressure ulcer of right heel, stage 4: ICD-10-CM Diagnosis Code_____

12. Acute lymphangitis of right toe: ICD-10-CM Diagnosis Code_____

13. Pemphigus vegetans: ICD-10-CM Diagnosis Code_____

14. Kyrle disease: ICD-10-CM Diagnosis Code_____

15. Freckles: ICD-10-CM Diagnosis Code_____

16. Pruritus ani: ICD-10-CM Diagnosis Code_____

17. Contact dermatitis due to nickel: ICD-10-CM Diagnosis Code_____

18. Bromhidrosis: ICD-10-CM Diagnosis Code_____

19. Keloid scar: ICD-10-CM Diagnosis Code_____

20. Hidradenitis suppurativa: ICD-10-CM Diagnosis Code_____

CODING PRACTICE CASES

Case 1

Betty Smith in seen in the office today for a skin rash she is concerned about. She reports that the rash is very itchy, and when she scratches it frequently it will start to bleed and does not seem to be healing. The physician examines Betty and finds that she has large dry, scaly red patches on her wrists and hands. The physician discusses the use of soap with Betty and asks if she has recently starting using a new soap or detergent. The physician diagnoses Betty as having eczema and discusses treatment options with her. What ICD-10-CM Code(s) are assigned?_____

Case 2

Martin Mower is seen in the emergency department for a swollen finger that is very sore and has pus oozing from it. Martin is a steelworker and reports that it has been difficult to complete his work and would like to get this taken care of. The emergency department physician examines Martin's left finger and determines that he has a severe case of cellulitis. The physician takes a sample of the wound drainage and sends it to the lab. The lab results reveal *Staphylococcus aureus*. The physician documents cellulitis due to *Staphylococcus aureus* and starts the patient on an antibiotic and warm compresses. He is to follow up in 7 days if the finger does not look better. What ICD-10-CM Code(s) are assigned?_____

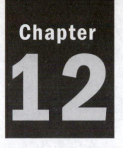
DISEASES OF THE MUSCULOSKELETAL SYSTEM AND CONNECTIVE TISSUE

SCAVENGER HUNT

Go to the JustCoding Website and read the following article:
http://www.justcoding.com/270313/icd10cmpcs-codes-for-musculoskeletal-system-include-greater-level-of-specificity

Discuss what is the most important element you took away from this article and the new ICD-10-CM Musculoskeletal system codes and why the content in this article will be helpful to you in your future career in coding.

APPLICATION ASSIGNMENT

Many times as a coder the physician's documentation will state the type of fracture. Research the following types of fractures and match up the correct fracture with the correct definition.

_____ 1. Greenstick
_____ 2. Transverse
_____ 3. Oblique
_____ 4. Comminuted
_____ 5. Buckle
_____ 6. Pathological
_____ 7. Stress

a. caused by a disease that weakens the bones
b. when the bone breaks into several pieces
c. also known as an impacted fracture, is one whose ends driven into each other; this is commonly seen in arm fractures in children
d. hairline crack
e. when the broken piece of bone is at a right angle to the bone's axis
f. when the break has a curved or sloped pattern
g. an incomplete fracture in which the bone is bent; this type occurs most often in children

CRITICAL THINKING

Select one of the Official Coding Guidelines that deals with Musculoskeletal System Coding from those in Section I. C.13.a–d (the official guidelines can be found at http://www.cdc.gov/nchs/data/icd/ICD10cmguidelines_2015%209_26_2014.pdf).

Describe what the guideline is saying and how we will use this in coding. Give a scenario example of when this guideline would be applied.

CODING CASES

1. Felty's syndrome of the left knee: ICD-10-CM Diagnosis Code
   _____

2. Gouty bursitis, right foot and ankle: ICD-10-CM Diagnosis
   Code_____

3. Bilateral primary osteoarthritis of the hips: ICD-10-CM Diagnosis
   Code_____

4. Ankylosis, right elbow: ICD-10-CM Diagnosis Code_____

5. Postural kyphosis, thoracic region: ICD-10-CM Diagnosis
   Code_____

6. Reiter's disease, left elbow: ICD-10-CM Diagnosis
   Code_____

7. Pneumococcal arthritis, left hand: ICD-10-CM Diagnosis
   Code_____

8. Juvenile arthritis, right wrist: ICD-10-CM Diagnosis
   Code_____

9. Kaschin-Beck disease, right knee: ICD-10-CM Diagnosis
   Code_____

10. Hemarthrosis, left shoulder: ICD-10-CM Diagnosis
    Code_____

11. Chronic osteomyelitis with draining sinus of the left humerus.
    ICD-10-CM Diagnosis Code_____

12. Calcaneal spur, right foot: ICD-10-CM Diagnosis Code_____

13. Infective arthritis: ICD-10-CM Diagnosis Code_____

14. Loose body in the left knee: ICD-10-CM Diagnosis
    Code_____

15. Age-related osteoporosis with current pathological fracture of the right
    forearm: ICD-10-CM Diagnosis Code_____

16. Primary gout of the right hip: ICD-10-CM Diagnosis
    Code_____

17. Pain in right thigh: ICD-10-CM Diagnosis Code_____

18. Rheumatoid polyneuropathy with rheumatoid arthritis of left hip:
    ICD-10-CM Diagnosis Code_____

19. Nontraumatic separation of muscle in the right arm: ICD-10-CM Diag-
    nosis Code_____

20. Lumbago with sciatica on the right side: ICD-10-CM Diagnosis
    Code_____

CODING PRACTICE CASES

Case 1

Today 37-year-old Beau Bobblee was seen today in the office for a sore arm. The physician examines Beau's arm which is very swollen, red, and hot to touch. The physician take a sample of the fluid and sends it to lab for review. The lab reports that the patient has *Streptococcus* A. The physician diagnoses the patient with infective myositis of the right upper arm due to Strep A. What ICD-10-CM Code(s) are assigned?_____

Case 2

Olive Ollinger was brought in today from the Skilled Nursing Facility in which she is a resident. Olive is complaining of pain in her left foot, and she is unable to bear any weight. Olive denies any accident or injury that might have injured her foot. Upon examination her foot is very swollen, and the physician orders an x-ray of the left foot, which reveals a pathological fracture of the left foot. What ICD-10-CM Code(s) are assigned?_____

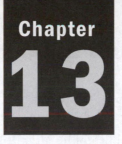
INJURY, POISONING, AND CERTAIN OTHER CONSEQUENCES OF EXTERNAL CAUSES

SCAVENGER HUNT

Go to AHIMA's website www.ahima and read the following article: http://library.ahima.org/xpedio/groups/public/documents/ahima/bok1_048533.hcsp?dDocName=bok1_048533

After you read the article, discuss one element in the article, either fracture coding, aftercare coding, injury, poisoning, or burn coding. Discuss what you learned about coding this type of condition in ICD-10-CM and how you will utilize this information in your future coding career.

APPLICATION ASSIGNMENT

Watch the following TedTalkVideo on "A new way to grow a bone." http://www.ted.com/talks/molly_stevens_a_new_way_to_grow_bone

Think about the types of injuries that we code that deal with bones, and discuss if you think this new treatment would be beneficial. Why or why not?

CRITICAL THINKING

Select one of the Official Coding Guidelines that deals with Injury, Poisoning and other consequences of external causes from those in Section I. C.19 a–g (the official guidelines can be found at http://www.cdc.gov/nchs/data/icd/ICD10cmguidelines_2015%209_26_2014.pdf).

Describe what the guideline is saying and how we will use this in coding. Give a scenario example of when this guideline would be applied.

CODING CASES

1. Current nonvenomous insect bite to the nose: ICD-10-CM Diagnosis Code and external cause code, when applicable_____

2. Splinter in right external ear: ICD-10-CM Diagnosis Code and external cause code, when applicable_____

3. Current traumatic rupture of left eardrum after patient fell off train while trying to board it: ICD-10-CM Diagnosis Code and external cause code, when applicable_____

4. Current superficial frostbite of right hand: ICD-10-CM Diagnosis Code and external cause code, when applicable_____

5. Current third-degree burn of lip after drinking hot coffee: ICD-10-CM Diagnosis Code and external cause code, when applicable_____

6. Dislocation of T6/T7 thoracic vertebra after patient fell out of tree today: ICD-10-CM Diagnosis Code and external cause code, when applicable_____

7. A 2-year old brought to the ER by his mother as he accidentally drank bay rum: ICD-10-CM Diagnosis Code and external cause code, when applicable_____

8. Patient seen for an open fracture of the shaft of the left humerus. The patient was kicked by a horse: ICD-10-CM Diagnosis Code and external cause code, when applicable_____

9. Patient came into the office for an abrasion of the scalp that she received from hitting her head on the coffee table today: ICD-10-CM Diagnosis Code and external cause code, when applicable_____

10. A 12-year-old has been seen for fractured ribs. The patient fractured three ribs on the right side today when he was struck by a baseball: ICD-10-CM Diagnosis Code and external cause code, when applicable_____

11. A 3-year-old was bitten by a dog today and presents to the ER with an open bite to the right index finger: ICD-10-CM Diagnosis Code and external cause code, when applicable_____

12. Patient is currently taking cyclosporin and presents to the ER for an adverse reaction to this medication: ICD-10-CM Diagnosis Code and external cause code, when applicable_____

13. Current first-degree burn of right palm from touching dry ice: ICD-10-CM Diagnosis Code and external cause code, when applicable_____

14. Patient brought in via ambulance after getting his arm caught in a band saw today. He has an amputation between the elbow and wrist of his right arm: ICD-10-CM Diagnosis Code and external cause code, when applicable_____

15. Patient was doing dishes tonight when she broke a glass and cut open her right index finger: ICD-10-CM Diagnosis Code and external cause code, when applicable_____

16. Patient was curling her hair today and accidentally burned her forehead with the curling iron: ICD-10-CM Diagnosis Code and external cause code, when applicable_____

17. Patient's boyfriend broke up with her so she took her mom's entire bottle of thyroid hormone replacement in a suicide attempt: ICD-10-CM Diagnosis Code and external cause code, when applicable_____

18. Patient sprained the deltoid ligament in her left ankle today when she accidentally tripped over a cat: ICD-10-CM Diagnosis Code and external cause code, when applicable_____

19. Patient fell off his nonmotorized scooter today and has a displaced transverse fracture of his right patella: ICD-10-CM Diagnosis Code and external cause code, when applicable_____

20. Patient seen today in the ER for an adverse reaction to her antihistamine medication: ICD-10-CM Diagnosis Code and external cause code, when applicable_____

 ## CODING PRACTICE CASES

Case 1

Joshua Johnson was up on a ladder today and he fell off. His mother called 911, and they told her to not let him move. The paramedics placed Joshua on a backboard and took him to the ED. The ED physician examined Joshua and determined that he suffered from a coccyx fracture and a stable burst fracture of his lumbar vertebra. What ICD-10-CM Code(s) are assigned?_____

Case 2

Molly Magdoline was boiling some water today and when she took the lid off the pan, the steam burned her. The physician examines Molly and determines that she has first-degree burns to her cheek and forehead and second-degree burns to her nose. What ICD-10-CM Code(s) are assigned?

_____

DISEASES OF THE CIRCULATORY SYSTEM

SCAVENGER HUNT

Go to the Justcoding website, and complete the circulatory system coding quiz http://www.justcoding.com/quiz/2629

There are five questions to the quiz. How did you do on the quiz the first try? How many times did it take you to get all five questions correct? What are the correct answers for each of the five questions? Of the five questions, which one was the hardest for you to find the correct code, and why?

APPLICATION ASSIGNMENT

Go to the MayoClinic website and watch the following video on the cardiovascular system. http://www.mayoclinic.org/diseases-conditions/heart-disease/multimedia/circulatory-system/vid-20084745

After you watched the video what was the most helpful part of this short video? How do you think you will utilize this knowledge in your future career in coding? Why, as a coder, is it important for us to fully understand how the cardiovascular system works?

CRITICAL THINKING

Select one of the Official Coding Guidelines that deals with Cardiovascular System Coding from those in Section I. C.9 a–e (the official guidelines can be found at http://www.cdc.gov/nchs/data/icd/ICD10cmguidelines_2015%209_26_2014.pdf).

Describe what the guideline is saying and how we will use this in coding. Give a scenario example of when this guideline would be applied.

CODING CASES

1. Crescendo angina: ICD-10-CM Diagnosis Code_____
2. Adhesive mediastinopericarditis: ICD-10-CM Diagnosis Code_____
3. Embolism of superficial veins of the right lower extremities: ICD-10-CM Diagnosis Code_____
4. Ataxia following cerebrovascular disease: ICD-10-CM Diagnosis Code_____

5. Atherosclerotic heart disease: ICD-10-CM Diagnosis Code_____

6. Sick sinus syndrome: ICD-10-CM Diagnosis Code_____

7. Raynaud's syndrome: ICD-10-CM Diagnosis Code_____

8. Dissection of renal artery: ICD-10-CM Diagnosis Code_____

9. Myocardial fibrosis: ICD-10-CM Diagnosis Code_____

10. Chronic venous hypertension with inflammation of left lower extremity: ICD-10-CM Diagnosis Code_____

11. Primary pulmonary hypertension: ICD-10-CM Diagnosis Code_____

12. Facial droop following cerebrovascular disease: ICD-10-CM Diagnosis Code_____

13. Ventricular fibrillation: ICD-10-CM Diagnosis Code_____

14. Chronic lymphangitis: ICD-10-CM Diagnosis Code_____

15. Aneurysm of iliac artery: ICD-10-CM Diagnosis Code_____

16. Septic myocarditis due to *Streptococcus B*: ICD-10-CM Diagnosis Code_____

17. Cardiac arrest: ICD-10-CM Diagnosis Code_____

18. Ischemic chest pain: ICD-10-CM Diagnosis Code_____

19. Acute embolism and thrombosis of left tibial vein: ICD-10-CM Diagnosis Code_____

20. Old myocardial infarction: ICD-10-CM Diagnosis Code_____

CODING PRACTICE CASES

Case 1

Arnold Anderson is a 65-year-old male patient who is brought to the ER today with severe chest pain that is radiating to his left arm. The physician orders a CPK, EKG, and stress test. After reviewing the results of the tests, the physician determines that the patient has had a STEMI involving the left circumflex artery. The patient was sent to University Hospital for cardiac consult. What ICD-10-CM Code(s) are assigned?_____

Case 2

Jeffrey Jones is a 75-year-old patient seen today for difficulty with speaking and memory. A CT scan is ordered, which revealed that the patient has a cerebral infraction from an embolism in the right carotid artery. The patient was also found to have hypertension and was started on a beta-blocker. What ICD-10-CM Code(s) are assigned?_____

DISEASES OF THE BLOOD AND BLOOD-FORMING ORGANS AND CERTAIN DISORDERS INVOLVING THE IMMUNE MECHANISM

SCAVENGER HUNT

Go to the Justcoding website, and complete the blood and blood-forming organs coding quiz: http://www.justcoding.com/quiz/2651

There are five questions to the quiz. How did you do on the quiz the first try? How many times did it take you to get all five questions correct? What are the correct answers for each of the five questions? Of the five questions, which one was the hardest for you to find the correct code for, and why?

APPLICATION ASSIGNMENT

Read the following article from the NIH on how anemia is diagnosed. Website is: http://www.nhlbi.nih.gov/health/health-topics/topics/anemia/diagnosis

As a coder, how might you utilize the information you found in this article? What was the most beneficial point discussed in this article for your future career in coding, and why?

CRITICAL THINKING

Select one of the Official Coding Guidelines that deals with General Coding Guidelines from those in Section I. B.1–18 (the official guidelines can be found at http://www.cdc.gov/nchs/data/icd/ICD10cmguidelines_2015%209_26_2014.pdf).

Describe what the guideline is saying and how we will use this in coding. Give a scenario example of when this guideline would be applied.

CODING CASES

1. Iron deficiency anemia due to secondary blood loss: ICD-10-CM Diagnosis Code_____

2. Prothrombin gene mutation: ICD-10-CM Diagnosis Code_____

3. Hyperimmunoglobulin E syndrome: ICD-10-CM Diagnosis Code_____

4. Acquired polycythemia: ICD-10-CM Diagnosis Code_____

5. Mediterranean anemia: ICD-10-CM Diagnosis Code_____

6. Hereditary hypogammaglobulinemia: ICD-10-CM Diagnosis Code_____

7. Von Willebrand's disease: ICD-10-CM Diagnosis Code_____

8. Hb- C disease: ICD-10-CM Diagnosis Code_____

9. Simple chronic anemia: ICD-10-CM Diagnosis Code_____

10. Sickle-cell thalassemia with acute chest syndrome: ICD-10-CM Diagnosis Code_____

11. Basophilia: ICD-10-CM Diagnosis Code_____

12. Pancytopenia: ICD-10-CM Diagnosis Code_____

13. Hereditary spherocytosis: ICD-10-CM Diagnosis Code_____

14. Thalassemia minor: ICD-10-CM Diagnosis Code_____

15. Activated protein C resistance: ICD-10-CM Diagnosis Code_____

16. Sarcoidosis of lung: ICD-10-CM Diagnosis Code_____

17. Elevated white blood cell count: ICD-10-CM Diagnosis Code_____

18. Atrophy of spleen: ICD-10-CM Diagnosis Code_____

19. Anemia: ICD-10-CM Diagnosis Code_____

20. Cryoglobulinemia purpura: ICD-10-CM Diagnosis Code_____

CODING PRACTICE CASES

Case 1

Calvin Conrad is being seen today for increased lethargy and fatigue. Calvin has colon cancer and has been receiving treatment for that for about 6 months. The physician examines Calvin and orders some labs. The results of the lab and examination reveal that Calvin has anemia due to carcinoma of the sigmoid colon. What is the correct ICD-10-CM Code(s) Assignment?_____

Case 2

Holly Hullbrook is being seen in the ER today for 3 days of extreme fatigue and lack of energy. Holly explains that she is very pale and just does not have the energy to get out of bed. She is not sure what is wrong. The physician examines Holly and completes a blood panel. Upon review of his findings, he diagnoses Holly with pancytopenia, anemia, and neutropenia. What is the correct ICD-10-CM Code(s) Assignment?_____

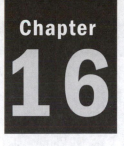
DISEASES OF THE RESPIRATORY SYSTEM

SCAVENGER HUNT

Go to the Justcoding website and Diseases of the Respiratory System coding quiz: http://www.justcoding.com/quiz/2497

There are five questions to the quiz. How did you do on the quiz the first try? How many times did it take you to get all five questions correct? What are the correct answers for each of the five questions? Of the five questions, which one was the hardest for you to find the correct code for, and why?

APPLICATION ASSIGNMENT

Go to Healthline, and watch the short video on Pneumonia: http://www.healthline.com/vpvideo/pneumonia

After you watched the video, what was the most helpful part of this short video? How do you think you will utilize this knowledge in your future career in coding? Why, as a coder, is it important for us to fully understand how the cardiovascular system works?

CRITICAL THINKING

Select one of the Official Coding Guidelines that deals with Respiratory System Coding from those in Section I. C.10 a–d (the official guidelines can be found at http://www.cdc.gov/nchs/data/icd/ICD10cmguidelines_2015%209_26_2014.pdf).

Describe what the guideline is saying and how we will use this in coding. Give a scenario example of when this guideline would be applied.

CODING CASES

1. Acute tonsillits: ICD-10-CM Diagnosis Code_____

2. Pneumonia due to *Klebsiella pneumoniae*: ICD-10-CM Diagnosis Code_____

3. Deviated nasal septum: ICD-10-CM Diagnosis Code_____

4. Simple chronic bronchitis: ICD-10-CM Diagnosis Code_____

5. Allergic rhinitis due to pollen: ICD-10-CM Diagnosis Code_____

6. Lymphangioleiomyomatosis: ICD-10-CM Diagnosis Code_____

7. Acute recurrent maxillary sinusitis: ICD-10-CM Diagnosis Code_____

8. Pneumonia due to *Streptococcus*, Group B: ICD-10-CM Diagnosis Code_____

9. Acute respiratory failure with hypoxia: ICD-10-CM Diagnosis Code_____

10. Byssinosis: ICD-10-CM Diagnosis Code_____

11. Atelectasis: ICD-10-CM Diagnosis Code_____

12. Enlargement of adenoids and tonsils: ICD-10-CM Diagnosis Code_____

13. Emphysema: ICD-10-CM Diagnosis Code_____

14. Cellulitis of the pharynx: ICD-10-CM Diagnosis Code_____

15. Acute bronchitis due to echovirus: ICD-10-CM Diagnosis Code_____

16. Severe persistent asthma with acute exacerbation: ICD-10-CM Diagnosis Code_____

17. Acute pansinusitis: ICD-10-CM Diagnosis Code_____

18. Pneumonia: ICD-10-CM Diagnosis Code_____

19. Acute abscess of vocal cords: ICD-10-CM Diagnosis Code_____

20. Acute laryngopharyngitis: ICD-10-CM Diagnosis Code_____

CODING PRACTICE CASES

Case 1

William Wolcolf is seen today in consultation by Dr. Smith, an ENT physician, for evaluation of a nasal deviation as well as sinus troubles. William complains that he has had difficulty breathing and thick mucous secretions in his sinuses for years. His primary care physician has tried a few different treatments on William, but nothing seems to work, so he was referred to Dr. Smith for evaluation. Dr. Smith examines William and completes a detailed history and physical. He determines that William has chronic maxillary sinusitis, chronic ethmoidal sinusitis, and a deviated nasal septum. He determines that surgery is needed. He discussed the benefits and risks of the surgery with William. What is the correct ICD-10-CM Code(s) Assignment? _____

Case 2

Helen Hunt is a 75-year-old patient who is a resident as Hollybrook Assisted Living Center. The aides at the assisted living center noticed that Helen has not been eating well, getting out of bed, or acting her normal perky self, so they brought her to the ED for examination. The ED physician speaks with Helen, who explains that she has been very tired, weak, has a cough, and feels like she has a fever. The vitals revealed a fever at 102.4°F. A sputum culture was collected, which showed mycoplasma pneumonia. The ED physician's diagnosis is pneumonia due to mycoplasma pneumonia. What is the correct ICD-10-CM Code(s) Assignment? _____

DISEASES OF THE NERVOUS SYSTEM AND SENSE ORGANS

SCAVENGER HUNT

Go to the Justcoding website and Diseases of the Nervous System coding quiz: http://www.justcoding.com/quiz/2610

There are five questions to the quiz. How did you do on the quiz the first try? How many times did it take you to get all five questions correct? What are the correct answers for each of the five questions? Of the five questions, which one was the hardest for you to find the correct code for, and why?

APPLICATION ASSIGNMENT

Go to WebMD and watch the video on Multiple Sclerosis: http://multiple-sclerosis.emedtv.com/multiple-sclerosis-video/the-nervous-system-video.html

After you watched the video, what was the most helpful part of this short video? How do you think you will utilize this knowledge in your future career in coding? Why, as a coder, is it important for us to fully understand how the cardiovascular system works?

CRITICAL THINKING

Select one of the Official Coding Guidelines that deals with Nervous System Coding from those in Section I. C.6 a–b (the official guidelines can be found at http://www.cdc.gov/nchs/data/icd/ICD10cmguidelines_2015%209_26_2014.pdf).

Describe what the guideline is saying and how we will use this in coding. Give a scenario example of when this guideline would be applied.

CODING CASES

1. Hemophilus meningitis: ICD-10-CM Diagnosis Code_____

2. Alzheimer disease with early onset: ICD-10-CM Diagnosis Code_____

3. Multiple sclerosis: ICD-10-CM Diagnosis Code_____

4. Migraine with aura, not intractable, without status migrainosus: ICD-10-CM Diagnosis Code_____

5. Congenital nonprogressive ataxia: ICD-10-CM Diagnosis Code_____

6. Intractable cyclical vomiting: ICD-10-CM Diagnosis Code_____

7. Middle cerebral artery syndrome: ICD-10-CM Diagnosis Code_____

8. Central pontine myelinolysis: ICD-10-CM Diagnosis Code_____

9. Ataxic cerebral palsy: ICD-10-CM Diagnosis Code_____

10. Cerebral abscess: ICD-10-CM Diagnosis Code_____

11. TIA: ICD-10-CM Diagnosis Code_____

12. Myotonic muscular dystrophy: ICD-10-CM Diagnosis Code_____

13. Dementia with Parkinsonism: ICD-10-CM Diagnosis Code_____

14. Alcoholic polyneuropathy: ICD-10-CM Diagnosis Code_____

15. Episodic tension-type headache: ICD-10-CM Diagnosis Code_____

16. Postencephalitic Parkinsonism: ICD-10-CM Diagnosis Code_____

17. Epilespy spasms, intractable, with status epilepticus: ICD-10-CM Diagnosis Code_____

18. Juvenile myoclonic epilepsy, intractable, without status epilepticus: ICD-10-CM Diagnosis Code_____

19. Familial tremor: ICD-10-CM Diagnosis Code_____

20. Blepharospasm: ICD-10-CM Diagnosis Code_____

CODING PRACTICE CASES

Case 1

Diane Denton is a secretary who has been having increased pain and numbness with tingling in her right hand. Her primary care physician examined her and felt that she needs to be seen by Dr. Johnson, an orthopedic surgeon. Dr. Johnson completes an examination and testing on Diane and determines she is suffering from Right Carpal Tunnel Syndrome. He recommends surgery and discusses the risks and benefits of surgery with Diane. What is the correct ICD-10-CM Code Assignment? _____

Case 2

Penelope Priddy is a 2-month-old female infant being seen today for obstructive hydrocephalus. Penelope was born prematurely and was immediately taken to surgery as an infant to insert a cerebral ventricle shunt for her hydrocephalus. Her follow-up visit today was good, and the physician determined her shunt is functioning fine. He asks for Penelope to return in 2 months, or as needed before. What is the correct ICD-10-CM Code Assignment? _____

MENTAL, BEHAVIORAL, AND NEURODEVELOPMENTAL DISORDERS

SCAVENGER HUNT

Read the following article from JustCoding: http://www.justcoding
.com/306188/identify-mental-disorder-details-for-icd10cm-coding

What was the most interesting part of the article, and why? When coding
mental disorders in the future, do you think that this information will be
beneficial to you? Why or why not? From all the mental disorders we have
in ICD-10-CM, which code do you think you might utilize more as a coder,
and why?

APPLICATION ASSIGNMENT

Go to Eating Disorders Online and watch the video "What is
Anorexia." http://www.eatingdisordersonline.com/videos/anorexia/
what-is-anorexia-nervosa-video

After watching the video, was there anything you learned about anorexia
that you did not know before? If so, what, and how will this information be
useful to you as a coder? Was there anything you learned about bulimia that
you did not know before? If so, what, and how will this information be useful
to you as a coder? Were the signs and symptoms mentioned in the video what
you expected? Why or why not, and how will you utilize these in coding?

CRITICAL THINKING

Select one of the Official Coding Guidelines that deals with Mental System
Coding from those in Section I. C.5 a–c (the official guidelines can be found
at: http://www.cdc.gov/nchs/data/icd/ICD10cmguidelines_2015%209_
26_2014.pdf).

Describe what the guideline is saying and how we will use this in coding.
Give a scenario example of when this guideline would be applied.

CODING CASES

1. Vascular dementia with aggressive behavior: ICD-10-CM Diagnosis Code_____

2. Bipolar disorder, current episode with mild depression: ICD-10-CM Diagnosis Code_____

3. Opioid dependence with intoxication with perceptual disturbance: ICD-10-CM Diagnosis Code_____

4. Vascular dementia with aggressive behavior: ICD-10-CM Diagnosis Code_____

5. Bulimia nervosa: ICD-10-CM Diagnosis Code_____

6. Presenile dementia: ICD-10-CM Diagnosis Code_____

7. Agoraphobia with panic disorder: ICD-10-CM Diagnosis Code_____

8. Cocaine abuse with cocaine-induced anxiety disorder: ICD-10-CM Diagnosis Code_____

9. Trichotillomania: ICD-10-CM Diagnosis Code_____

10. Transient tic disorder: ICD-10-CM Diagnosis Code_____

11. Inhalant abuse: ICD-10-CM Diagnosis Code_____

12. Borderline personality disorder: ICD-10-CM Diagnosis Code_____

13. Alcohol abuse: ICD-10-CM Diagnosis Code_____

14. Asperger's syndrome: ICD-10-CM Diagnosis Code_____

15. Primary insomnia: ICD-10-CM Diagnosis Code_____

16. Cannabis dependence, in remission: ICD-10-CM Diagnosis Code_____

17. Anxiety reaction: ICD-10-CM Diagnosis Code_____

18. Childhood ADHD: ICD-10-CM Diagnosis Code_____

19. Abuse of steroids: ICD-10-CM Diagnosis Code_____

20. Alcohol dependence with alcohol induced sleep disorder: ICD-10-CM Diagnosis Code_____

CODING PRACTICE CASES

Case 1

Nannette Nudge is a 21-year-old personal trainer who is very athletic. Nannette was running yesterday when she passed out and was brought to the ER. The ER physician examined Nannette and determined that she has a very low body weight and is concerned about her dietary intake. After discussing her daily caloric intake the ER physician determines that Nannette is suffering from restricting anorexia nervosa. The ER physician refers Nannette to Dr. Would, a psychiatrist, as well as Jan Bates, a dietician, to get her caloric intake where it needs to be. What is the correct ICD-10-CM Code Assignment? _____

Case 2

Robert Roundup is seen today by Dr. Would in a severe panic attack. Dr. Would has been treating Robert for a little over a year trying to control his disorder with medication. Today he returns complaining that the medication is not working, as he is under a lot of concern and feels a panic attack frequently. Robert is also suffering from Adjustment Disorder with depressed mood after the recent loss of his mother, who was his main caregiver. What is the correct ICD-10-CM Code Assignment?_____

DISEASES OF THE EYE
AND ADNEXA

SCAVENGER HUNT

Go to the Justcoding website and Diseases of the Eye and Adnexa coding quiz: http://www.justcoding.com/quiz/2550

There are five questions to the quiz. How did you do on the quiz the first try? How many times did it take you to get all five questions correct? What are the correct answers for each of the five questions? Of the five questions, which one was the hardest for you to find the correct code for, and why?

APPLICATION ASSIGNMENT

Go to the Glaucoma.org website and watch the video on glaucoma.

http://www.glaucoma.org/glaucoma/video-what-is-glaucoma.php

What did you learn about glaucoma that you did not previously know? What treatments did you learn about that you did not know about before? How will this information help as you are coding glaucoma? When coding glaucoma what will the coder need to know, and how will your new knowledge from this video be beneficial during your code assignment for glaucoma?

CRITICAL THINKING

Select one of the Official Coding Guidelines that deals with Disease of the Eye and Adnexa Coding from those in Section I. C.7 a (the official guidelines can be found at http://www.cdc.gov/nchs/data/icd/ICD10cmguidelines_2015%209_26_2014.pdf).

Describe what the guideline is saying and how we will use this in coding. Give a scenario example of when this guideline would be applied.

CODING CASES

1. Anterior scleritis of the right eye: ICD-10-CM Diagnosis Code_____

2. Primary cyst of pars plana, left eye: ICD-10-CM Diagnosis Code_____

3. Bilateral aphakia: ICD-10-CM Diagnosis Code_____

4. Ghost vessels in both eyes: ICD-10-CM Diagnosis Code_____

5. Both eyes have hypertensive retinopathy: ICD-10-CM Diagnosis Code_____

6. Iridodialysis: ICD-10-CM Diagnosis Code_____

7. Conjunctival granuloma, left eye: ICD-10-CM Diagnosis Code_____

8. Preglaucoma, left eye: ICD-10-CM Diagnosis Code_____

9. Degenerative myopia of the right eye: ICD-10-CM Diagnosis Code_____

10. Cyst of ora serrata, left eye: ICD-10-CM Diagnosis Code_____

11. Snow blindness: ICD-10-CM Diagnosis Code_____

12. V pattern alternating exotropia: ICD-10-CM Diagnosis Code_____

13. Senile cataract: ICD-10-CM Diagnosis Code_____

14. Descemetocele, right eye: ICD-10-CM Diagnosis Code_____

15. Vitreoretinal dystrophy: ICD-10-CM Diagnosis Code_____

16. Recurrent pterygium, left eye: ICD-10-CM Diagnosis Code_____

17. An 11-week-old with retinopathy of prematurity in the left eye: ICD-10-CM Diagnosis Code_____

18. Choroidal rupture, right eye: ICD-10-CM Diagnosis Code_____

19. Bullous keratopathy, right eye: ICD-10-CM Diagnosis Code_____

20. Chronic conjunctivitis, left eye: ICD-10-CM Diagnosis Code_____

CODING PRACTICE CASES

Case 1

David Doldoor presents to the opthlamologist for evaluation of vision, as David recently failed the eye test at the drivers' license office. The physician examined David and tested both the right and left eyes. The physician discovered that David has vertical strabismus of the left eye and bilateral astigmatism. What is the correct ICD-10-CM Code Assignment? _____

Case 2

Eugina Evans is seen today for treatment of her glaucoma. Eugina has had glaucoma for about 3 years and has been treating it with eye drops. She is out of eye drops and is returning to have her glaucoma checked and refill her eye drop prescription. Dr. Miles reviewed Eugina's history and performed a detailed examination on her eyes. He determined that her chronic angle-closure glaucoma of the right eye is in the mild stage and is responding well to the eye drops and refills her prescription telling Eugina to return in 6 months to check her pressure and eyes again. What is the correct ICD-10-CM Code Assignment? _____

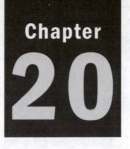
DISEASES OF THE EAR AND THE MASTOID PROCESS

 ## SCAVENGER HUNT

Go to the Justcoding website and Diseases of the Ear and the Mastoid Process coding quiz: http://www.justcoding.com/quiz/2452

There are five questions to the quiz. How did you do on the quiz the first try? How many times did it take you to get all five questions correct? What are the correct answers for each of the five questions? Of the five questions, which one was the hardest for you to find the correct code for, and why?

APPLICATION ASSIGNMENT

Go to Science Daily, and watch the video "Brainstem implants help deaf children hear." http://www.sciencedaily.com/videos/8eea586be22d461ca563ca5cef30e1cb.htm

What did you find most interesting about this video? As a future coder why is understanding new procedures for disease and condition important? How will the knowledge gained from this video help you in your future coding career?

CRITICAL THINKING

Select one of the Official Coding Guidelines that deals with Selection of the Principal Diagnosis from those in Section II. A–K (the official guidelines can be found at http://www.cdc.gov/nchs/data/icd/ICD10cmguidelines_2015%209_26_2014.pdf).

Describe what the guideline is saying and how we will use this in coding. Give a scenario example of when this guideline would be applied.

 ## CODING CASES

1. Boil of external ear: ICD-10-CM Diagnosis Code_____

2. Bilateral conductive hearing loss: ICD-10-CM Diagnosis Code_____

3. Bilateral otitis media: ICD-10-CM Diagnosis Code_____

4. Left ear with tympanosclerosis: ICD-10-CM Diagnosis Code_____

5. Ear disorder of the right ear: ICD-10-CM Diagnosis Code_____

6. Acute mastoiditis in the left ear: ICD-10-CM Diagnosis Code_____

7. Right ear has acute actinic otitis externa: ICD-10-CM Diagnosis Code_____

8. Diplacusis, right ear: ICD-10-CM Diagnosis Code_____

9. Polyp of right middle ear: ICD-10-CM Diagnosis Code_____

10. Cochlear otosclerosis of the right ear: ICD-10-CM Diagnosis Code_____

11. Ménière disease in both ears: ICD-10-CM Diagnosis Code_____

12. Bilateral suppurative otitis media: ICD-10-CM Diagnosis Code_____

13. Bilateral chronic otitis externa: ICD-10-CM Diagnosis Code_____

14. Diffuse cholesteatosis in the left ear: ICD-10-CM Diagnosis Code_____

15. Ear pain in the left ear: ICD-10-CM Diagnosis Code_____

16. Labyrinthitis of the right ear: ICD-10-CM Diagnosis Code_____

17. Chronic petrositis, left ear: ICD-10-CM Diagnosis Code_____

18. Tinnitus: ICD-10-CM Diagnosis Code_____

19. Presbycusis: ICD-10-CM Diagnosis Code_____

20. Right ear has impacted cerumen: ICD-10-CM Diagnosis Code_____

CODING PRACTICE CASES

Case 1

Madison Monroe is a 3-year-old with recurrent ear infections who is brought to the same-day surgery suite for a bilateral tympanostomy with ventilating tube placement. The surgery went fine, and the postoperative diagnosis is bilateral chronic serous otitis media. What is the correct ICD-10-CM Code Assignment? _____

Case 2

Wilbur Wilson is brought to the ED today by his wife. She is concerned that he is deaf, as he never hears what she is saying. The ED physician completes a detailed history and examination on Wilbur, and after a few tests he determines that Wilbur has a perforation of the tympanic membrane in the right ear and bilateral impacted cerumen. The physician removes the cerumen and refers Wilbur to Dr. Wills, an ENT specialist, to examine the perforation. What is the correct ICD-10-CM Code Assignment? _____

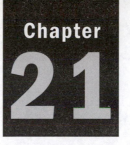

CERTAIN INFECTIOUS AND PARASITIC DISEASES

SCAVENGER HUNT

Go to the Justcoding website and Diseases of the Nervous System coding quiz http://justcoding.com/quiz/2523

There are five questions to the quiz. How did you do on the quiz the first try? How many times did it take you to get all five questions correct? What are the correct answers for each of the five questions? Of the five questions, which one was the hardest for you to find the correct code for, and why?

APPLICATION ASSIGNMENT

Go to SepsisAlliance.org, and watch one of the videos on Sepsis: http://www .sepsisalliance.org/resources/video/

What video did you select, and why did you select that video? After you watch the video what new information did you learn about Sepsis. How will you utilize this information in your future coding career? Why is coding sepsis so important and how can you remember the difference between sepsis, severe sepsis and septic shock?

CRITICAL THINKING

Select one of the Official Coding Guidelines that deals with Certain Infectious and Parasitic Diseases Coding from those in Section I. C. 1. a–e (the official guidelines can be found at http://www.cdc.gov/nchs/data/icd/ ICD10cmguidelines_2015%209_26_2014.pdf).

Describe what the guideline is saying and how we will use this in coding. Give a scenario example of when this guideline would be applied.

CODING CASES

1. Adenoviral enteritis: ICD-10-CM Diagnosis Code_____
2. Meningococcal meningitis: ICD-10-CM Diagnosis Code_____
3. Infestation of head lice: ICD-10-CM Diagnosis Code_____
4. Cryptosporidiosis: ICD-10-CM Diagnosis Code_____
5. Swimmer's itch: ICD-10-CM Diagnosis Code_____

6. Cat-scratch fever: ICD-10-CM Diagnosis Code_____

7. Toxoplasma myocarditis: ICD-10-CM Diagnosis Code_____

8. Conjunctivitis due to adenovirus: ICD-10-CM Diagnosis Code_____

9. Latent syphilis: ICD-10-CM Diagnosis Code_____

10. TB of the lung: ICD-10-CM Diagnosis Code_____

11. Sepsis due to *Streptococcus* A: ICD-10-CM Diagnosis Code_____

12. Acarine dermatitis: ICD-10-CM Diagnosis Code_____

13. Acute hepatitis C with hepatic coma: ICD-10-CM Diagnosis Code_____

14. Candidal onychia: ICD-10-CM Diagnosis Code_____

15. Whooping cough due to *Bordetella pertussis*: ICD-10-CM Diagnosis Code_____

16. Tinea blanca: ICD-10-CM Diagnosis Code_____

17. Cutaneous anthrax: ICD-10-CM Diagnosis Code_____

18. *Echinococcus granulosus* infection of liver: ICD-10-CM Diagnosis Code_____

19. TSS due to *Staphylococcus aureus*: ICD-10-CM Diagnosis Code_____

20. Bubonic plague: ICD-10-CM Diagnosis Code_____

CODING PRACTICE CASES

Case 1

Ethan Embroy is a 28-month-old child who has been doing well until recently. Ethan has had a severe cough for 5 days. His primary care physician is concerned, as the mother is also reporting that Ethan has not been eating well and is very tired and weak. The primary care physician admits Ethan to the pediatric floor for workup. A chest x-ray was ordered, which shows that Ethan has pneumonia. His sputum cultures grew *Bordetella pertussis*. The physician started Ethan on antibiotics, and the discharge diagnosis is whooping cough due to *Bordetella pertussis* with pneumonia. What is the correct ICD-10-CM Code Assignment?_____

Case 2

Roger Randolph is seen in the dermatologist's office today for a skin growth. Roger is HIV positive. The dermatologist biopsies Roger's skin growth, which shows Kaposi's sarcoma. The diagnosis is Kaposi's sarcoma of the skin due to HIV disease. What is the correct ICD-10-CM Code Assignment?_____

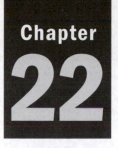

DISEASES OF THE GENITOURINARY SYSTEM

⬤ SCAVENGER HUNT

Go to AHIMA's website and read the following article: https://newsletters.ahima.org/newsletters/ICDTen/2011/October/reproductive.html

Read the article, and discuss what you found most beneficial from this article. What new information did you learn about coding diseases of the genitourinary system? The article discusses how the female/male reproductive and urinary systems work together. As coders will we be coding conditions from both often? Why or why not? As a new coder what was the most valuable piece of this article for you, and why?

⬤ APPLICATION ASSIGNMENT

Go to About.com, and watch the video on treating urinary tract infections: http://video.about.com/menshealth/How-to-Treat-a-Urinary-Tract-Infection.htm

After you watch the video, discuss what the most valuable piece of new information was that you learned. Why is this information helpful, and how will you use this in your future coding career? When coding a UTI, what documentation will the coder need to look for, and where can this information be found?

⬤ CRITICAL THINKING

Select one of the Official Coding Guidelines that deals with Genitourinary Coding from those in Section I. C.14 a (the official guidelines can be found at http://www.cdc.gov/nchs/data/icd/ICD10cmguidelines_2015%209_26_2014.pdf).

Describe what the guideline is saying and how we will use this in coding. Give a scenario example of when this guideline would be applied.

CODING CASES

1. Chronic obstructive pyelonephritis: ICD-10-CM Diagnosis Code_____

2. Megaloureter: ICD-10-CM Diagnosis Code_____

3. Priapism: ICD-10-CM Diagnosis Code_____

4. Lateral cystocele: ICD-10-CM Diagnosis Code_____

5. Diffuse cystic mastopathy of the right breast: ICD-10-CM Diagnosis Code_____

6. Urethral fistula: ICD-10-CM Diagnosis Code_____

7. Mild chronic kidney disease: ICD-10-CM Diagnosis Code_____

8. Leukoplakia of cervix: ICD-10-CM Diagnosis Code_____

9. Solitary acquired cyst of kidney: ICD-10-CM Diagnosis Code_____

10. Kraurosis of penis: ICD-10-CM Diagnosis Code_____

11. Acute salpingitis and oophoritis: ICD-10-CM Diagnosis Code_____

12. Simple cyst of the ovary: ICD-10-CM Diagnosis Code_____

13. Balkan endemic nephropathy: ICD-10-CM Diagnosis Code_____

14. Postmenopausal bleeding: ICD-10-CM Diagnosis Code_____

15. Vaginal polyp: ICD-10-CM Diagnosis Code_____

16. Page kidney: ICD-10-CM Diagnosis Code_____

17. Cyst of Bartholin's gland: ICD-10-CM Diagnosis Code_____

18. Mastodynia: ICD-10-CM Diagnosis Code_____

19. Torsion of testis: ICD-10-CM Diagnosis Code_____

20. Hydronephrosis: ICD-10-CM Diagnosis Code_____

CODING PRACTICE CASES

Case 1

Mark Miller is seen today by Dr. Jensen, a urologist, to have his penis examined. Mark is an uncircumcised male and has been experiencing a discharge. Upon examination, Mark's penis is very red and swollen. The physician determines that Mark has phimosis and balanoposthitis and recommends that he receive a circumcision to remedy the situation. Dr. Jensen discusses the benefits and risks of the procedure with Mark. What is the correct ICD-10-CM Code Assignment?_____

Case 2

Crissy Calloway has been trying to conceive for 1 year without any success. She presents to the hospital today for a hysterosalpingogram. The physician reviews the results of the hysterosalpingogram and finds that Crissy has infertility due to severe pelvic peritoneal adhesions that are blocking both of her fallopian tubes. The physician recommends that Crissy undergo a laparoscopic lysis of these adhesions. The benefits and risks of the procedure were discussed with Crissy. What is the correct ICD-10-CM Code Assignment?_____

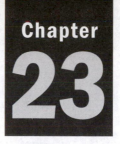

PREGNANCY, CHILDBIRTH, AND THE PUERPERIUM

SCAVENGER HUNT

Go to AHIMA's website and read the following article: http://library .ahima.org/xpedio/groups/public/documents/ahima/bok1_047548 .hcsp?dDocName=bok1_047548

Read the article, and discuss what you found most beneficial. What new information did you learn about coding pregnancy, childbirth, and the puerperium? The article discusses how some codes need to be identified by trimesters. Explain what a trimester is and the gestational period for each one. As coders, what do you think will be some common conditions you will code from this section? As a new coder what was the most valuable piece of this article for you, and why?

APPLICATION ASSIGNMENT

Go to WebMD and watch the video on hysterectomies: http://www.webmd .com/women/video/hysterectomy

After you watch the video, discuss what the most valuable piece of new information was that you learned. Why is this information helpful, and how will you use this in your future coding career? Why is it important for coders to understand surgeries and how they are completed?

CRITICAL THINKING

Select one of the Official Coding Guidelines that deals with Pregnancy, Childbirth and the Puerperium Coding from those in Section I. C.15 a–r (the official guidelines can be found at http://www.cdc.gov/nchs/data/icd/ ICD10cmguidelines_2015%209_26_2014.pdf).

Describe what the guideline is saying and how we will use this in coding. Give a scenario example of when this guideline would be applied.

CODING CASES

1. Molar pregnancy: ICD-10-CM Diagnosis Code_____
2. Abnormal glucose complicating pregnancy. Patient is currently 17 weeks along: ICD-10-CM Diagnosis Code_____

3. Patient is at 34 weeks gestation and is being seen for gestational edema: ICD-10-CM Diagnosis Code_____

4. Mammary abscess associated with lactation: ICD-10-CM Diagnosis Code_____

5. Patient testing positive for syphilis, and the physician wants it under control before she delivers the baby; she is at 12 weeks gestation: ICD-10-CM Diagnosis Code_____

6. UTI following incomplete spontaneous abortion: ICD-10-CM Diagnosis Code_____

7. Postpartum fibrinolysis: ICD-10-CM Diagnosis Code_____

8. Patient delivered 2 days ago and is now coming back in for severe pain. The physician determines she has cervicitis following the delivery and prescribes an antibiotic: ICD-10-CM Diagnosis Code_____

9. Galactorrhea: ICD-10-CM Diagnosis Code_____

10. Pregnancy complicated by preexisting essential hypertension at week 22: ICD-10-CM Diagnosis Code_____

11. A 30-year-old female seen today to discuss smoking cessation as she is currently 8 weeks pregnant and would like to quit smoking, as she is not gaining the weight her physician would like: ICD-10-CM Diagnosis Code_____

12. Patient just received an ultrasound at 13 weeks and is carrying triplets. Her primary care physician is transferring her care to an OB/GYN that can deal with multiple babies: ICD-10-CM Diagnosis Code_____

13. Primary agalactia: ICD-10-CM Diagnosis Code_____

14. Hemorrhoids in the puerperium: ICD-10-CM Diagnosis Code_____

15. Cardiac arrest following termination of pregnancy: ICD-10-CM Diagnosis Code_____

16. A 23-year-old female currently at 32 weeks gestation who is complaining of varicose veins in her lower extremity: ICD-10-CM Diagnosis Code_____

17. Herpes gestation is at 37 weeks: ICD-10-CM Diagnosis Code_____

18. Disruption of cesarean delivery wound: ICD-10-CM Diagnosis Code_____

19. Patient is currently being seen at 12 weeks gestation for anemia that is complicating her pregnancy: ICD-10-CM Diagnosis Code_____

20. Supervision of pregnancy, 1st trimester, in a patient with a history of infertility: ICD-10-CM Diagnosis Code_____

CODING PRACTICE CASES

Case 1

Jamie Jones is a 25-year-old gravida 2 para 1 who presents to labor and delivery in active labor at 39½ weeks. Jamie is admitted to labor suite 1, and the physician is alerted. Jamie delivers a healthy female liveborn 7 lbs 9 oz. 19 inches long without any complications. What is the correct ICD-10-CM Code Assignment?_____

Case 2

Wendy Waller is a 30-year-old patient being seen today at 10 weeks gestation for excessive vomiting. Wendy reports that she is unable to keep anything down. The physician determines that Wendy has mild hyperemesis gravidarum and gives her a prescription to help with the nausea and vomiting. He tells Wendy to call his office if the condition continues. What is the correct ICD-10-CM Code Assignment?_____

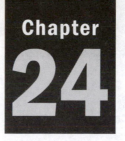

CERTAIN CONDITIONS ORIGINATING IN THE PERINATAL PERIOD

SCAVENGER HUNT

Go to the Justcoding website and Diseases of the Nervous System coding quiz: http://www.justcoding.com/quiz/2679

There are five questions to the quiz. How did you do on the quiz the first try? How many times did it take you to get all five questions correct? What are the correct answers for each of the five questions? Of the five questions, which one was the hardest for you to find the correct code for, and why?

APPLICATION ASSIGNMENT

Go to the National Heart, Lung and Blood Institute, and read the following article on Infant Respiratory Distress Syndrome: http://www.nhlbi.nih.gov/health/health-topics/topics/rds/treatment

After you read the article, discuss what you found most beneficial. What new information did you learn about coding infant ARDS? The article discusses some different treatments for ARDS. Explain why it is important for coders to understand these treatments. As a new coder, what was the most valuable piece of this article for you, and why?

CRITICAL THINKING

Select one of the Official Coding Guidelines that deals with Perinatal Conditions Coding from those in Section I. C.16 a–g (the official guidelines can be found at http://www.cdc.gov/nchs/data/icd/ICD10cmguidelines_2015%209_26_2014.pdf).

Describe what the guideline is saying and how we will use this in coding. Give a scenario example of when this guideline would be applied.

CODING CASES

1. Newborn small for gestational age weighting 1750 grams: ICD-10-CM Diagnosis Code_____

2. RH isoimmunization of newborn: ICD-10-CM Diagnosis Code_____

3. Mild hypothermia of newborn: ICD-10-CM Diagnosis Code_____

4. Stage 1 necrotizing enterocolitis in newborn: ICD-10-CM Diagnosis Code_____

5. Bilious vomiting of newborn: ICD-10-CM Diagnosis Code_____

6. Kernicterus: ICD-10-CM Diagnosis Code_____

7. Failure to thrive in newborn: ICD-10-CM Diagnosis Code_____

8. Premature infant born at 32 weeks: ICD-10-CM Diagnosis Code_____

9. Gray baby syndrome: ICD-10-CM Diagnosis Code_____

10. Neonatal cardiac failure: ICD-10-CM Diagnosis Code_____

11. Congenital hydrocele: ICD-10-CM Diagnosis Code_____

12. Neonatal jaundice due to bleeding: ICD-10-CM Diagnosis Code_____

13. Floppy baby syndrome: ICD-10-CM Diagnosis Code_____

14. Neonatal erythema toxicum: ICD-10-CM Diagnosis Code_____

15. Rupture of liver due to birth injury: ICD-10-CM Diagnosis Code_____

16. Wilson-Mikity syndrome: ICD-10-CM Diagnosis Code_____

17. Congenital rubella syndrome: ICD-10-CM Diagnosis Code_____

18. Newborn with meconium staining: ICD-10-CM Diagnosis Code_____

19. Polycythemia neonatorum: ICD-10-CM Diagnosis Code_____

20. Bruising of scalp due to birth injury: ICD-10-CM Diagnosis Code_____

CODING PRACTICE CASES

Case 1

Jordan Jensen is a 1-day-old liveborn male infant who was delivered via cesarean delivery yesterday. Jordan weighed 8 lbs 8 oz and was 21 inches long. Today he developed pale skin and severe swelling of the body. Test were run, and it was determined that Jordan suffered from hemolytic disease due to an ABO isoimmunization. A blood transfusion was given to treat the infant. What is the correct ICD-10-CM Code Assignment?_____

Case 2

Mackenzie Miller is a 3-year-old seen today in the office for evaluation of Erb's palsy. Mackenzie has Erb's palsy from a birth trauma. She has been going to a physical therapist to help and continues home exercises. The physician is interested in performing Botox injections to help rebalance the muscles, and the mother will discuss this with the father and make a follow-up appointment at a later date. What is the correct ICD-10-CM Code Assignment?_____

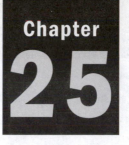

CONGENITAL MALFORMATIONS, DEFORMATIONS, AND CHROMOSOMAL ABNORMALITIES

SCAVENGER HUNT

Go to the Justcoding website and Diseases of the Congenital Malformations of the respiratory system coding quiz http://www.justcoding.com/quiz/2942

There are five questions to the quiz. How did you do on the quiz the first try? How many times did it take you to get all five questions correct? What are the correct answers for each of the five questions? Of the five questions, which one was the hardest for you to find the correct code for, and why?

APPLICATION ASSIGNMENT

Go to Detroit Medical Center and watch the video on repairing a cleft palate: http://www.dmc.org/VideoLibrary/ShowVideo .aspx?Library=1&VideoID=110

What did you find most shocking about this video? What information did you find to be the most valuable as you think about coding a cleft palate repair? Discuss why as a coder the visual picture of a procedure is beneficial in coding. Finally, what did you find most interesting in the video, and why?

CRITICAL THINKING

Select one of the Official Coding Guidelines that covers Outpatient Services from those in Section I. C.IV A–Q (the official guidelines can be found at http://www.cdc.gov/nchs/data/icd/ICD10cmguidelines_2015%209_26_2014.pdf).

Describe what the guideline is saying and how we will use this in coding. Give a scenario example of when this guideline would be applied.

CODING CASES

1. Coarctation of aorta: ICD-10-CM Diagnosis Code_____
2. Hemicephaly: ICD-10-CM Diagnosis Code_____
3. Choanal atresia: ICD-10-CM Diagnosis Code_____
4. A 2-week-old infant who is tongue tied: ICD-10-CM Diagnosis Code_____

5. Webbed toes on both feet: ICD-10-CM Diagnosis Code_____

6. Harnold-Chiaris syndrome, type IV: ICD-10-CM Diagnosis Code_____

7. Ectopic right testis: ICD-10-CM Diagnosis Code_____

8. Ebstein's anomaly: ICD-10-CM Diagnosis Code_____

9. Congenital blind loop syndrome: ICD-10-CM Diagnosis Code_____

10. Congenital funnel chest: ICD-10-CM Diagnosis Code_____

11. Aplasia of the right eye: ICD-10-CM Diagnosis Code_____

12. Congenital torsion of ovary: ICD-10-CM Diagnosis Code_____

13. Gottic web of larynx: ICD-10-CM Diagnosis Code_____

14. Crouzon's disease: ICD-10-CM Diagnosis Code_____

15. Cleft uvula: ICD-10-CM Diagnosis Code_____

16. Duplication of ureter: ICD-10-CM Diagnosis Code_____

17. A 2-month-old with annular pancreas: ICD-10-CM Diagnosis Code_____

18. Marcus Gunn's syndrome: ICD-10-CM Diagnosis Code_____

19. Congenital bronchomalacia: ICD-10-CM Diagnosis Code_____

20. Atrial septal defect: ICD-10-CM Diagnosis Code_____

CODING PRACTICE CASES

Case 1

Bradley Benson was born 2 days ago at the community hospital but now needs neonatal intensive care, so he was transferred from the community hospital to the Children's hospital. He is admitted to the Children's hospital with congestive heart failure with a congenital interatrial septal defect. What is the correct ICD-10-CM Code Assignment?_____

Case 2

Carson Cambridge is a 6-month-old male referred to the ENT office for evaluation of Carson's reflux esophagitis. The physician determines that Carson has esophageal web with esophageal spasm in addition to the reflux esophagitis. Dr. Bradley discusses the prognosis and treatment options with Carson's parents. What is the correct ICD-10-CM Code Assignment?_____

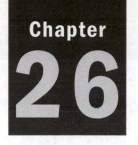

Chapter

26

SCAVENGER HUNT

Go to the AHIMA website and look at the following document: http://library.ahima.org/xpedio/groups/public/documents/ahima/bok1_038084.hcsp?dDocName = bok1_038084

Review this comparison between ICD-9 and ICD-10, and discuss why you think the change to ICD-10 was needed. Do you think that ICD-10 is a superior coding system when compared to ICD-9? Why or why not? What do you think the extra characters in ICD-10-CM codes allow for that ICD-9 did not?

CRITICAL THINKING ACTIVITIES

Go to HCPro.com and read the following article: http://www.hcpro.com/HOM-293035-7200/ICD9-vs-ICD10-Similarities-and-differences.html

What do you think is beneficial about the new ICD-10 system when compared to the ICD-9 system? What do you think some of the similarities of the two systems are? If you could change anything else between ICD-9 and ICD-10, what would it be, and why?

APPLICATION ASSIGNMENT

Using the ICD-10-CM Codes provided for the following scenarios go to www.icd10data.com and convert the following ICD-10 codes into ICD-9-CM Codes.

1. Blepharitis of the left lower eyelid: ICD-10-CM: H01.005

2. Carcinoma of the tail of the pancreas: ICD-10-CM: C25.2

3. Rapid heartbeat: ICD-10-CM Diagnosis Code R00.0

4. Healthy newborn baby check for a newborn 12 days old: ICD-10-CM: Z00.111

5. A 7-year-old who fell off his skateboard today: ICD-10-CM: V00.131A

6. Acute appendicitis with generalized peritonitis: ICD-10-CM: K35.2

7. Type I diabetes mellitus with mild nonproliferative diabetic retinopathy with macular edema: ICD-10-CM:

8. Plaque psoriasis: ICD-10-CM: L40.0

9. Felty's syndrome of the left knee: ICD-10-CM: M05.062

10. Current nonvenomous insect bite to the nose: ICD-10-CM: S00.37XA, W57.XXXA

11. Crescendo angina: ICD-10-CM: I20.0

12. Iron deficiency anemia due to secondary blood loss: ICD-10-CM: D50.0

13. Acute tonsillitis: ICD-10-CM: J03.90

14. Hemophilus meningitis: ICD-10-CM: G00.0

15. Vascular dementia with aggressive behavior: ICD-10-CM: F01.51

16. Anterior scleritis of the right eye: ICD-10-CM: H15.011

17. Boil of external ear: ICD-10-CM: H60.00

18. Adenoviral enteritis: ICD-10-CM: A08.2

19. Chronic obstructive pyelonephritis: ICD-10-CM: N11.1

20. Molar pregnancy: ICD-10-CM: O02.0

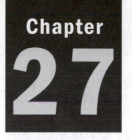

ICD-9-CM BODY SYSTEM CODING

SCAVENGER HUNT

Go to the CDC website and read the following document: http://www.cdc .gov/nchs/icd/icd10cm_pcs_background.htm

After you read the document, based on the list of difference between the ICD-9-CM Procedure Coding Set and ICD-10-PCS, which one do you think will be most beneficial, and why? Do you think that ICD-10-PCS is a superior coding system when compared to ICD-9-CM Volume III? Why or why not? How do you think the quality of data will be improved with ICD-10-PCS versus ICD-9-CM Volume III?

CRITICAL THINKING ACTIVITIES

Go to World Health Organization and read the following article: http://www .who.int/classifications/icd/revision/icd11faq/en/

With ICD-11 on the horizon for the rest of the world, what does that mean for us in the United States as we are still waiting for the implementation of ICD-10? Why is ICD-10 needed before one can transition to ICD-11? What would happen if a country tried to go from ICD-9 to ICD-11? Do you think the United States will be ready for ICD-11 by the potential 2017 WHO implementation date? Why or why not? As a coder, why is it important to stay abreast of changes the WHO is making?

APPLICATION ASSIGNMENT

Using the ICD-10-CM Codes provided for the following scenarios, go to www.icd10data.com and convert the following ICD-10 Codes into ICD-9-CM Codes.

1. Corbus' disease: ICD-10-CM Diagnosis Code N48.1
2. Neoplasm of the breast: ICD-10-CM Diagnosis Code D49.3
3. Hyperglycemia: ICD-10-CM Diagnosis Code R73.9
4. Patient who is being seen for bereavement of a family member: ICD-10-CM Diagnosis Code Z63.4
5. RH isoimmunization of newborn: ICD-10-CM Diagnosis Code P55.0
6. Sialolithiasis: ICD-10-CM Diagnosis Code K11.5
7. Bartter's syndrome: ICD-10-CM Diagnosis Code E26.81

8. Allergic dermatitis due to dog dander: ICD-10-CM Diagnosis Code L23.81

9. Gouty bursitis, right foot and ankle: ICD-10-CM Diagnosis Code M10.071

10. Coarctation of aorta: ICD-10-CM Diagnosis Code Q25.1

11. Adhesive mediastinopericarditis: ICD-10-CM Diagnosis Code I31.0

12. Prothrombin gene mutation: ICD-10-CM Diagnosis Code D68.52

13. Pneumonia due to *Klebsiella pneumoniae*: ICD-10-CM Diagnosis Code J15.0

14. Alzheimer disease with early onset: ICD-10-CM Diagnosis Code G30.0

15. Bipolar disorder, current episode with mild depression: ICD-10-CM Diagnosis Code F31.30

16. Primary cyst of pars plana, left eye: ICD-10-CM Diagnosis Code H21.342

17. Bilateral conductive hearing loss: ICD-10-CM Diagnosis Code H90.0

18. Meningococcal meningitis: ICD-10-CM Diagnosis Code A39.0

19. Megaloureter: ICD-10-CM Diagnosis Code N28.82

20. Abnormal glucose complicating pregnancy. Patient is currently 17 weeks along: ICD-10-CM Diagnosis Code O99.810

INTRODUCTION TO CPT PROCEDURE CODING

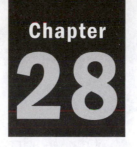

Chapter
28

SCAVENGER HUNT

Go to Quizlet and practice the six sections of the CPT Coding Manual- https://quizlet.com/1973577/cptdefinition-of-the-six-cpt-sections-flash-cards/

Why is it important to understand all six of these as a coder? Which section is the smallest? Which section is the biggest? Which section do you think you will use the most as a coder, and why? Which section do you think you will use the least as a coder, and why?

APPLICATION ASSIGNMENT

Go to Quizlet, and practice the CPT Introduction flashcard: https://quizlet .com/19641733/cpt-introduction-flash-cards/

Which of these were the easiest to remember, and which were the hardest? Why? As a future coder, why it is important that you have all these terms and concepts? What are some ways you can ensure that you master these terms and concepts?

CRITICAL THINKING

Go to the Coding Pirates website, and click on the Basic Steps to CPT Coding under the video link at: http://www.thecodingpirates.com/ basic-steps-to-cpt-coding/

After you watch the video, what was the most beneficial part of the video, and why? What did you learn from the video that you did not know before? How will you use the knowledge gained from this video in your future coding career?

CODING CASES

What is the main term in each of the following scenarios that you would look up in the CPT index?

1. Surgical thoracoscopy with chemical pleurodesis
2. Implantation of bone conduction in the right ear
3. Intracapsular cataract extraction
4. Biopsy of the spinal cord
5. Complete mastoidectomy
6. Complicated pyelotomy
7. Radical resection of an abdominal wall tumor
8. Pharynx myotomy
9. Second order abdominal arterial selective catheterization
10. Surgical laparoscopy with radical hysterectomy
11. Established patient seen for office visit
12. Lengthening of tendon in the left finger
13. Blepharoptosis repair of the right eye
14. Incision and drainage of large bladder abscess
15. Inpatient consultation
16. Missed abortion first trimester
17. Esophageal motility study with perfusion
18. Macrodactylia repair of three digits
19. Intravenous hydration
20. Inpatient hospital discharge day

INTRODUCTION TO HCPCS CODING

⬤ SCAVENGER HUNT

Go to the MedicalCoding website and complete the HCPCS coding quiz: http://www.justcoding.com/quiz/2041

There are five questions to the quiz. How did you do on the quiz the first try? How many times did it take you to get all five questions correct? What are the correct answers for each of the five questions? Of the five questions, which one was the hardest for you to find the correct code for, and why?

⬤ APPLICATION ASSIGNMENT

Go to the CMS's website and read the following article: http://www.cms.gov/Medicare/Coding/MedHCPCSGenInfo/HCPCS_Coding_Questions.html

After you read the article, discuss the differences between HCPCS Level I and HCPCS Level II. Discuss why we have both levels. The article also mentions the OPPS system. Why are HCPCS important in the OPPS system? As a future coder why must you understand the OPPS system and how coding is utilized for this system?

⬤ CRITICAL THINKING

Go to the CMS website and to the following pdf guide on how to use the Noridian's HCPCS search function: https://www.dmepdac.com/docs/search/dmecs_guide.pdf

Follow the instructions in the pdf file. Once you get to Search for HCPCS information,

"Using a HCPCS Code Search 1. Enter a code into the HCPCS Code field. 2. Click GO or the Enter button on the keyboard."

Enter 10 HCPCS supplies, medicines, or durable medical equipment, such as wheelchair, catheter, orthotic, Pitocin (or other medications), and list the 10 HCPCS codes that you found. How helpful do you think it will be to have this tool? Do you think coders are using this Noridian PDAC? Why or why not? Do you think in the future you would utilize this tool? Why or why not?

⬤ CODING CASES

Assign the correct HCPCS codes to the following cases:

1. A 65-year-old who was supplied with an air pressure mattress to help with decubitus ulcers. What is the correct HCPCS code(s)?

2. A 45-year-old with DVT who received a full-length style 30-44 gradient compression stocking. What is the correct HCPCS code(s)?

3. Newborn infant born today at 27 weeks was transferred via ambulance from the birth hospital to the Children's Hospital for treatment of extreme prematurity. What is the correct HCPCS code(s)?

4. Patient seen in the office with an eye injury. He was given a sterile eye pad. What is the correct HCPCS code(s)?

5. A 64-year-old seen today for an echocardiogram and was given an injection of contrast material prior to the echo. What is the correct HCPCS code(s)?

6. A 74-year-old received parenteral nutrition administration kits for three days. What is the correct HCPCS code(s)?

7. A 36-year-old who received an implantable breast prosthesis. What is the correct HCPCS code(s)?

8. A 55-year-old male who has emphysema and was supplied an adult oxygen tent. What is the correct HCPCS code(s)?

9. A 65 year-old patient is here today for intragastric hypothermia using gastric freezing. What is the correct HCPCS code(s)?

10. Family planning for an 18-year-old patient with a diaphragm for contraceptive use. What is the correct HCPCS code(s)?

11. Patient receives two ostomy rings. What is the correct HCPCS code(s)?

12. Beta Smith was prescribed 50 mg of oral azathioprine for chronic postrheumatic arthropathy. What is the correct HCPCS code(s)?

13. A 12-year-old patient was in a bike accident and received a nonadjustable flexible cervical foam collar. What is the correct HCPCS code(s)?

14. Patient received 1 million units of Interferon, alfa-2B, recombinant. What is the correct HCPCS code(s)?

15. A 76-year-old COPD patient was supplied an oxygen and water vapor enriching system with heated delivery. What is the correct HCPCS code(s)?

16. The oxygen company delivered Mary Sue a cylinder tank carrier for her wheelchair. What is the correct HCPCS code(s)?

17. A 35-year-old received 25 mg of Clozapine. What is the correct HCPCS code(s)?

18. A 53-year-old received a prosthetic eye after removal of an eye melanoma. What is the correct HCPCS code(s)?

19. Sign language services for 45 minutes. What is the correct HCPCS code(s)?

20. A 4-year-old who received a single-power solid seat pediatric wheelchair. What is the correct HCPCS code(s)?

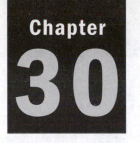

CPT MODIFIERS

SCAVENGER HUNT

Go to the CMS website and read the following article: http://www
.wpsmedicare.com/j8macpartb/resources/modifiers/modifierintro.shtml

What was the most helpful tip you learned about using modifiers from this
article? What is the difference between Level I and Level II modifiers, and
why do we need to know both of these as a coder?

APPLICATION ASSIGNMENT

Match the following modifiers with their description

_____	23	bilateral procedure
_____	26	reduced services
_____	32	preoperative management only
_____	33	professional component
_____	47	distinct procedural services
_____	50	mandated services
_____	51	staged procedure
_____	52	multiple procedures
_____	53	discontinued procedure
_____	54	surgical care only
_____	55	decision for surgery
_____	57	anesthesia by surgeon
_____	57	preventative services
_____	58	unusual anesthesia
_____	59	postoperative management only

CRITICAL THINKING

Go to the WPS website and look at the modifier fact sheets: http://www
.wpsmedicare.com/j5macpartb/resources/modifiers/

Select one of the modifier fact sheets. Read what the sheet states, and discuss
which modifier fact sheet you selected and the summary of what it said. As
a coder, why is it important to understand the proper use of modifiers? What
might happen if coders do not use modifiers appropriately? Finally, discuss
what new information you learned about the modifier you selected and how
you will utilize this in your future coding career.

CODING CASES

Which modifier is applicable to the following scenarios?

1. Bilateral tympanostomy. What is the correct modifier?

2. Bunionectomy of right great toe. What is the correct modifier?

3. Insurance company is requiring a second opinion for a surgical procedure. What is the correct modifier?

4. Patient being seen for her annual wellness mammogram. What is the correct modifier?

5. Nephrostomy of the left kidney. What is the correct modifier?

6. CABG performed by Dr. Smith and Dr. Lewis acting as cosurgeons. What is the correct modifier?

7. Dr. Petty was called into the OR to assist Dr. Jones in a complicated intra-abdominal trauma patient from MVA. What is the correct modifier?

8. Dr. Smith was asked to read the C-spine report taken at Bear River Hospital. What is the correct modifier?

9. Betty Jo had an EGD and colonoscopy during the same operative session. What is the correct modifier?

10. Cataract removal of the right eye. What is the correct modifier?

11. Joe Dreyser was in the OR getting an ORIF for a left femur fracture when he went into cardiac arrest, and the procedure was aborted. What is the correct modifier?

12. A 2-year-old is getting a cavity fixed in the same-day surgery suite under general anesthesia. What is the correct modifier?

13. Fracture repair of the left great toe. What is the correct modifier?

14. The physician ordered a repeat CBC on the same day. What is the correct modifier?

15. Patient was seen in the ER for bronchitis. Was given a Z-Pak and sent home. On the way home he was involved in an MVA and is now back in the ER for whiplash. What is the correct modifier?

16. Stent in the right coronary artery. What is the correct modifier?

17. Patient was admitted to SDS suite for hernia repair. When the anesthesiologist came to visit the patient, he discovered the patient had eaten breakfast before arriving at the hospital, so the patient is sent home and will reschedule surgery. What is the correct modifier?

18. Patient fractured her left ring finger after accidentally slamming it in a car door. What is the correct modifier?

19. Patient was seen in the office for a mole removal. After the physician successfully removed the mole, the patient was complaining of a sore throat. The physician examined patient's throat and ordered a strep culture. What is the correct modifier?

20. Blepharoplasty of the left lower eyelid. What is the correct modifier?

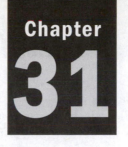
EVALUATION AND MANAGEMENT SERVICES

SCAVENGER HUNT

Go to the ACEP website, and read the following article: http://www.acep
.org/content.aspx?id=30416

What did you find most helpful about this article? From the questions and
answers provided, is there one that you were not aware of? If so, which was it?
How will you utilize this information in your future coding career?

APPLICATION ASSIGNMENT

Go to Quizlet, and practice the steps for E/M code assignment: https://quizlet
.com/1858882/steps-for-cpt-coding-flash-cards/

Which step in E/M code assignment is the most difficult for a coder, and
why? As a new coder how can you ensure you are following the correct steps?
Discuss how a new patient and an established patient impact these steps.

CRITICAL THINKING

Go to E-Med Tools website, and read the following article: http://e-medtools.
com/Medicare_Coding_Tool.html

What did you find most beneficial about this article. Do you think the E/M
cheat sheet will be a useful resource as a coder? Why or why not? How often
do you think a coder might use a similar sheet? Click on the Trailblazer
Health E&M Worksheet. Do you think that this will be a useful resource
as a coder? Why or why not? Of the two, which sheet did you find easier to
understand?

CODING CASES

1. Sadie Silverston is a 5-month-old new patient brought to the office
   today by her mother for diaper rash. The physician completes a history
   and exam, and the medical decision making is straightforward with the
   prescription of ointment to heal the diaper rash. What is the correct
   E/M code assigned?

2. Darryl Dievins was seen in the ER as she was exposed to poison oak
   while camping. The ER physician completes an expanded problem-
   focused exam, history and decision making were low. What is the correct E/M code assigned?

3. Betty Bilds is seen today for an initial office consultation for evaluation of her multiple sclerosis. Her current medication is not working, and her MS symptoms are getting worse. The physician performs a comprehensive history and examination. What is the correct E/M code assigned?

4. Initial hospital visit for Olivia Olson, who is a 1-day-old premature female born with extreme prematurity and will be transferred to the Neonatal Intensive Care Unit. What is the correct E/M code assigned?

5. Subsequent hospital visit for 46-year-old male with resolving acute colitis. The physician will be discharging the patient on the following day. What is the correct E/M code assigned?

6. Bob Butler is an established patient seen in the office today for a temperature of 102°F and diarrhea for 5 days. An expanded focused history and examination were completed. What is the correct E/M code assigned?

7. An 18-year-old female is seen by a gynecologist today for the first time for her annual GYN examination. They discussed contraception, and the physician took a complete history and physical. What is the correct E/M code assigned?

8. Dr. Smith sees Paul Puttolki today, who is an established patient with advanced glaucoma, at the patient's home. His family members express concern to the physician as Paul will not let any health care workers come in and help him, and they are concerned about his safety. The physician completes an expanded problem-focused history. The exam includes an examination of the HEENT and other symptomatic organ systems. The physician discusses the possibility of a skilled nursing facility for the patient if he is refusing home health. The family will discuss their options and let the physician know. What is the correct E/M code assigned?

9. A 65-year-old male is brought in to the ER at 12:08 with chest pain and goes into cardiac arrest. Lifesaving measures and critical care are provided to the patient for 48 minutes, but he expired at 12:56. What is the correct E/M code assigned?

10. Dr. Hart was asked to perform a surgical consult on Braiden Bernard, who is a 3-week-old male infant who was born with a hole in his heart. Dr. Hart completes a comprehensive history and exam on Braiden with a confirmation of the need for immediate surgery to fix his heart defect. What is the correct E/M code assigned?

11. 23-year-old Molly Magdolie is seen today by Dr. Sanderson for evaluation of her tennis elbow. Molly is usually treated by Dr. James, but he felt she needed an orthopedic consultation for her elbow and sent her to Dr. Sanderson for an evaluation. Dr. Sanderson completes an expanded problem-focused history and exam, and he decides to splint her for 4 weeks and have her return to evaluation at that time. What is the correct E/M code assigned?

12. Jeffrey Jackson was admitted for a routine hernia repair. His surgery was uncomplicated. Jeffrey has now developed a rash on his back, and his surgeon asked for Dr. Hill, a dermatologist, to review Jeffrey's rash. Dr. Hill performs a problem-focused history and exam and determines it is an allergy and prescribed an antihistamine. What is the correct E/M code assigned?

13. Maggie Miller is seen by Dr. Johnston today for the first time for complaints of a severe headache and runny nose. Dr. Johnston performs an expanded problem-focused exam and determines that her symptoms are due to her allergies and prescribes some medication to alleviate the symptoms. What is the correct E/M code assigned?

14. Dr. Anderson is seeing Ruth Rutska today in the Shady Acres Skilled Nursing Facility for the first time, as she was just admitted yesterday. Ruth has COPD and CHF and just underwent a TKA. Dr. Anderson performs a detailed history and examination on Ruth. What is the correct E/M code assigned?

15. Dr. Congy reviews the INR for anticoagulant management for an outpatient visit of John James, who is taking warfarin. What is the correct E/M code assigned?

16. Robert Randolph is seen today for a smoking cessation counseling visit that lasted 15 minutes. What is the correct E/M code assigned?

17. Bradley Benson is a 16-year-old seen today for the first time by Dr. Crackle for depression. Bradley explains to Dr. Crackle that he has been bullied at school, doesn't feel like he is worth anything, and doesn't really see any reason to live. Dr. Crackle completes a comprehensive history and discusses the bullying issues further with Bradley as well as his home situation and relationships with family and friends. Dr. Crackle discusses the need to have someone talk to him about any issues and urges Bradley to confide more in his parents. Dr. Crackle completes a comprehensive examination, determines that Bradley is suffering from severe depression, and is going to start him on Prozac to see if that will help reduce the negative thoughts and low self-worth that Bradley seems to feel. Dr. Crackle asks Bradley's mom to bring him back in 2 weeks to evaluate if the medication is working. What is the correct E/M code assigned?

18. Dr. Hiati performs a disability visit on Ralph Jones that includes his height, weight, blood pressure, and a basic life disability examination. What is the correct E/M code assigned?

19. Jamie Jillston, a nurse practitioner, meets with Helga Holdstein to explain and discuss her advance directives. Jamie helps Helga complete the forms and spend 25 minutes with the patient. What is the correct E/M code assigned?

20. Colby Cittro is an 11-year-old boy who is on a competitive swim team. The last couple of days his right ear has been bothering him, so Colby's mom took him into his family practice physician, Dr. Beck, to see what is going on. Dr. Beck completed a problem-focused history and exam and determines that Colby is suffering from swimmer's ear. What is the correct E/M code assigned?

CODING PRACTICE

Case 1

Mike Metro is a 48-year-old male who just moved to the area from out of state. He received a referral from the ER to see Dr. Baller, a primary care physician, for an annual wellness visit. Dr. Baller completes a comprehensive history and exam. He discusses with Mike the risk factors associated with his age and gender as well as orders a series of labs to evaluate Mike's overall health. What is the correct E/M code assigned?

Case 2

Tommy Tiller, a 12-year-old, was brought to the ER by his mother after Tommy wrecked on his bicycle and is now unable to bear any weight on his left leg. The ER physician completes an expanded problem-focused history and examination. He determines that Tommy has a sprained left ankle. He places Tommy in a brace and asks him to stay off his ankle for 1 week and follow up if it isn't getting better. What is the correct E/M code assigned?

MEDICINE SERVICES

SCAVENGER HUNT

Go to the Justcoding website, and Vaccine coding quiz: http://justcoding
.com/quiz/2637

There are five questions to the quiz. How did you do on the quiz the first
try? How many times did it take you to get all five questions correct? What
are the correct answers for each of the five questions? Of the five questions,
which one was the hardest for you to find the correct code, and why?

APPLICATION ASSIGNMENT

Go to Quizlet, and practice the CPT medicine flashcards: https://quizlet
.com/11030330/medical-coding-guideline-review-flash-cards/

Which of these were the easiest to remember, and which of these were the
hardest, and why? As a future coder, why it is important that you know all
these terms and concepts? What are some ways you can ensure that you master these terms and concepts?

CRITICAL THINKING

Go to the AAFP website, and read the following article on coding immuniza-
tions: http://www.aafp.org/practice-management/payment/coding/admin.html

What was the most important thing you learned from this article, and why?
How do you see yourself utilizing this information in your future as a coder?
What type of coder do you think will utilize vaccine codes more than others,
and why?

CODING CASES

1. Intermittent positive pressure breathing therapy for a newborn infant.
    What is the correct CPT code assigned?

2. A 6-year-old receiving a DTaP immunization. What is the correct CPT
    code(s) assigned?

3. Insertion of Swan-Ganz flow-directed catheter for monitoring. What is
    the correct CPT code assigned?

4. Awake and drowsy EEG performed without any complications. What is the correct CPT code assigned?

5. Allergy testing for wheat, eggs and animal dander using percutaneous methods of scratch, puncture, and prick. What is the correct CPT code assigned?

6. Services for allergen immunotherapy in physician's office with two or more injections with provision of allergenic extract by physician. What is the correct CPT code assigned?

7. Chemotherapy administration, intravenous, push technique. What is the correct CPT code assigned?

8. Photochemotherapy, ultraviolet B, tar. What is the correct CPT code assigned?

9. Violet Viper is seen today for physical therapy to develop strength and endurance for a patient who has been bedridden for 2 months. Violet received 30 minutes of therapy. What is the correct CPT code assigned?

10. Muscle testing of the entire body, including the hands. What is the correct CPT code assigned?

11. Mark Mason received individual biofeedback training, face-to-face for 30 minutes. What is the correct CPT code assigned?

12. CPR for 30 minutes with external cardioversion. What is the correct CPT code assigned?

13. A 6-year-old seen for speech audiometry threshold with speech recognition. What is the correct CPT code assigned?

14. A 67-year-old male seen for cardiovascular stress testing using maximal treadmill exercise with continuous electrocardiographic monitoring with physician supervision and interpretation and report. What is the correct CPT code assigned?

15. Inhalation bronchial challenge testing with antigens. What is the correct CPT code assigned?

16. A 4-year-old seen today for vaccination against measles, mumps, rubella, and varicella. What is the correct CPT code assigned?

17. A 19-year-old with chiropractic spinal manipulation in five regions. What is the correct CPT code assigned?

18. Patient seen for orthotics fitting and training of her upper extremity. The visit was 30 minutes. What is the correct CPT code assigned?

19. Patient seen by physical therapy for wheelchair propulsion training. The visit lasted 15 minutes. What is the correct CPT code assigned?

20. Dr. Smith had to provide medical testimony in court for a malpractice case. What is the correct CPT code assigned?

CODING PRACTICE

Case 1

Carly Jo was brought to the ER by her mother, as she suspected Carly Jo took some pills out of a Tylenol bottle. The physician administered Ipecac to induce vomiting and continued observing Carly until her stomach was emptied. What is the correct CPT code assigned?

Case 2

Billy Basin is a 63-year-old male with malignant lesions of his left arm. He is seen today for photodynamic therapy. Dr. Jill performs phototherapy by external application of light and activation of photosensitive drugs to destroy the malignant lesions. What is the correct CPT code assigned?

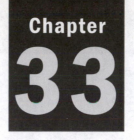

OVERVIEW OF SURGERY CODING

SCAVENGER HUNT

Go to Advance for Health Information, and read the article CPT Surgery Coding Guidelines Must Be Reviewed: http://health-information.advance-web.com/Article/CPT-Surgery-Coding-Guidelines—Must-Be-Reviewed.aspx

What was the most important concept you learned after reading this article? Discuss why, as a coder, it is imperative that the coding guidelines are understood. What can happen if the coder does not fully understand the coding guidelines?

APPLICATION ASSIGNMENT

Go to Quizlet, and practice the CPT Introduction to surgeries flashcard: https://quizlet.com/24533989/surgery-guidelines-and-general-surgery-list-flash-cards/

Which of these were the easiest to remember, and which of these were the hardest, and why? As a future coder why it is important that you know all these terms and concepts? What are some ways you can ensure that you master these terms and concepts?

CRITICAL THINKING

Go to the JustCoding website, and read the following article: http://www.justcoding.com/271641/identify-important-concepts-for-general-surgery-coding

What was the most important aspect of the article for you as you start your coding career? How did the section on examining the documentation impact you, and how important was this reminder? What happens if a coder does not fully examine the documentation? Discuss why understanding the approach is so important and what can happen if the approach is not fully understood by the coder.

CODING CASES

1. Drainage of the right knee. What is the correct CPT code assigned?
2. Exploration of the duodenum. What is the correct CPT code assigned?
3. Partial colectomy. What is the correct CPT code assigned?
4. Cesarean delivery. What is the correct CPT code assigned?
5. Brain debridement. What is the correct CPT code assigned?
6. Coronoidectomy of the TM joint. What is the correct CPT code assigned?
7. Septaldermatoplasty. What is the correct CPT code assigned?
8. Drainage of the left elbow bursa. What is the correct CPT code assigned?
9. Brachial artery embolectomy. What is the correct CPT code assigned?
10. Excision of the hippocampus. What is the correct CPT code assigned?
11. Anterior colporrhaphy with insertion of mesh. What is the correct CPT code assigned?
12. Artificial intra-uterine insemination. What is the correct CPT code assigned?
13. Central shunt. What is the correct CPT code assigned?
14. Diagnostic colonoscopy. What is the correct CPT code assigned?
15. Biopsy of the left cornea. What is the correct CPT code assigned?
16. Cystourethroscopy of the bladder with evacuation of a clot. What is the correct CPT code assigned?
17. Right breast capsulotomy. What is the correct CPT code assigned?
18. Left ankle arthrodesis. What is the correct CPT code assigned?
19. Thermal destruction of hemorrhoids. What is the correct CPT code assigned?
20. Bifrontal craniotomy. What is the correct CPT code assigned?

CODING PRACTICE

Case 1
Miley Miller is seen today in the same-day surgery suite for eye repair. Miley is prepped, draped, and anesthetized and taken to the OR. The physician completes a blepharoplasty of the right upper eyelid. What is the correct CPT code assigned?

Case 2
Carol Calloway is seen today in the same-day surgery suite for evaluation of a cyst on her left breast. Carol is prepped, draped, and anesthetized and taken to the OR. The physician completes an aspiration of a cyst in her left breast. What is the correct CPT code assigned?

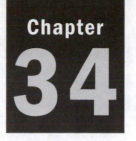
ANESTHESIA PROCEDURES

SCAVENGER HUNT

Go to the Medical Coding website, and complete the Anesthesia coding quiz: http://www.medicalcoding123.com/2012/09/anesthesia-questions.html

There are five questions to the quiz. How did you do on the quiz the first try? How many times did it take you to get all five questions correct? What are the correct answers for each of the five questions? Of the five questions, which one was the hardest for you to find the correct code, and why?

APPLICATION ASSIGNMENT

Match the correct P modifier description to the correct P modifier

_____	1. P1	a. Patient with mild systemic disease
_____	2. P2	b. A declared brain-dead patient whose organs are being removed for donor purposes
_____	3. P3	c. Normal healthy patient
_____	4. P4	d. Moribund patient who is not expected to survive without the operation
_____	5. P5	e. Patient with severe systemic disease
_____	6. P6	f. Patient with severe systemic disease that is a constant threat to life

CRITICAL THINKING

Go to the AAPC website, and read the PPT on Ten Steps to Coding Anesthesia Services: http://static.aapc.com/a3c7c3fe-6fa1-4d67-8534-a3c9c8315fa0/e0bdf19e-6a7c-4179-9300-8acc467f224e/d8a4f0fd-938b-458d-a1cd-0f1e2966e6d6.pdf

After you read each of the 71 slides, which one did you find the most beneficial, and why? Why is understanding the bundled codes important? What can happen if a coder does not understand the bundled codes? Why is the qualifying circumstance important for a coder to understand? What can happen if a coder is not aware of the qualifying circumstances or how to utilize these?

CODING CASES

1. Anesthesia for a percutaneous liver biopsy. What is the correct CPT Anesthesia code assigned?

2. Anesthesia for a heart transplant in a patient who is not expected to live without the surgery. What is the correct CPT Anesthesia code assigned?

3. Anesthesia for a total knee replacement. What is the correct CPT Anesthesia code assigned?

4. Anesthesia for a salivary gland biopsy. What is the correct CPT Anesthesia code assigned?

5. Anesthesia for vaginal delivery. What is the correct CPT Anesthesia code assigned?

6. Anesthesia for a pneumocentesis. What is the correct CPT Anesthesia code assigned?

7. Anesthesia for repair of a cleft palate. What is the correct CPT Anesthesia code assigned?

8. Anesthesia for craniectomy with evacuation of a hematoma. What is the correct CPT Anesthesia code assigned?

9. Anesthesia for TURP. What is the correct CPT Anesthesia code assigned?

10. Anesthesia for direct coronary artery bypass grafting with pump oxygenator. What is the correct CPT Anesthesia code assigned?

11. Anesthesia for a total hip arthroplasty. What is the correct CPT Anesthesia code assigned?

12. Anesthesia for extracorporeal shock wave lithotripsy with water bath. What is the correct CPT Anesthesia code assigned?

13. Anesthesia for insertion of a permanent transvenous pacemaker. What is the correct CPT Anesthesia code assigned?

14. Anesthesia for an arthroscopic osteotomy of humerus. What is the correct CPT Anesthesia code assign?

15. Anesthesia for a panniculectomy. What is the correct CPT Anesthesia code assigned?

16. Anesthesia for repair of a ruptured Achilles tendon. What is the correct CPT Anesthesia code assigned?

17. Anesthesia for an amniocentesis. What is the correct CPT Anesthesia code assigned?

18. Anesthesia for a corneal transplant. What is the correct CPT Anesthesia code assigned?

19. Physiological support for harvesting of organs from brain-dead patient. What is the correct CPT Anesthesia code assigned?

20. Anesthesia for a cardiac catheterization. What is the correct CPT Anesthesia code assigned?

CODING PRACTICE

Case 1

Robert Richards is seen in the ER for severe swelling and pain in his left leg. The physician orders some tests and workups and diagnoses him with an embolism in his left lower leg. The ER physician calls in surgery, who immediately takes Robert to the OR for an embolectomy of his left lower leg. What is the correct CPT Anesthesia code assigned?

Case 2

Semone Simon is a 26-year-old female in labor at 39½ completed weeks. Semone is Gravida 2 Para 1 and is here for a repeat C-section. Semone was taken to the OR, where a successful low cervical cesarean section was performed without difficulty. A healthy 7 lb. 12 oz. female infant who was 20 inches long was delivered without any complications. What is the correct CPT Anesthesia code assigned?

DIGESTIVE SYSTEM PROCEDURES

SCAVENGER HUNT

Go to the Justcoding website and Digestive System coding quiz: http://www .justcoding.com/quiz/2837

There are five questions to the quiz. How did you do on the quiz the first try? How many times did it take you to get all five questions correct? What are the correct answers for each of the five questions? Of the five questions, which one was the hardest for you to find the correct code, and why?

APPLICATION ASSIGNMENT

Anatomy Labeling. Please identify the structures of the digestive system by filling in the blanks:

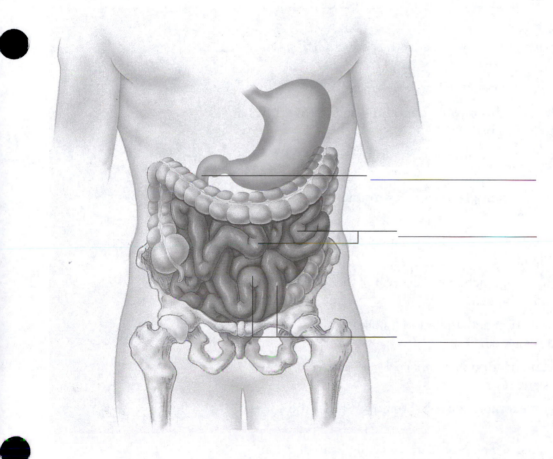

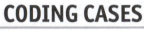

CRITICAL THINKING

Go to MedlinePlus, and watch the video on colonoscopy via the following link: http://www.orlive.com/broward-health/videos/what-is-a-colonoscopy?UPDATEAPP=false&VIEW=displayPageNLM

After you watch the video what was the most interesting part? As a coder, is it important to visually understand what you are coding? Why or why not? How do you think this video will be beneficial to you in your future coding career?

CODING CASES

1. Complicated removal of an embedded foreign body from the vestibule of the mouth. What is the correct CPT code assigned?

2. Dilation of esophagus using a guide wire. What is the correct CPT code assigned?

3. Laparoscopic partial colectomy with anastomosis and coloproctostomy. What is the correct CPT code assigned?

4. Bilateral posterior vestibuloplatsy. What is the correct CPT code assigned?

5. Gastrojejunostomy with vagotomy. What is the correct CPT code assigned?

6. Biopsy of lip. What is the correct CPT code assigned?

7. Diagnostic ileostomy through stoma with brushing and washings. What is the correct CPT code assigned?

8. Transrectal drainage of a pelvic abscess. What is the correct CPT code assigned?

9. Selective vagotomy with pyloroplasty with gastrostomy. What is the correct CPT code assigned?

10. Proctosigmoidoscopy with decompression of a volvulus. What is the correct CPT code assigned?

11. Esophagotomy, thoracic approach, with removal of foreign body. What is the correct CPT code assigned?

12. Diagnostic gastric intubation and aspiration for acid analysis. What is the correct CPT code assigned?

13. Flexible EGD with band ligation of esophageal varices. What is the correct CPT code assigned?

14. Transanal approach for excision of a rectal tumor. What is the correct CPT code assigned?

15. Drainage of parotid abscess. The procedure was complicated. What is the correct CPT code assigned?

16. Closure of intestinal cutaneous fistula. What is the correct CPT code assigned?

17. Laparotomy with biopsy of stomach. What is the correct CPT code assigned?

18. ERCP with multiple biopsies. What is the correct CPT code assigned?

19. Total abdominal colectomy with ileostomy. What is the correct CPT code assigned?

20. A 10-year-old who had a tonsillectomy and adenoidectomy. What is the correct CPT code assigned?

CODING PRACTICE

Case 1

Becker Bennett is seen in the OR today for an EGD. The patient is prepped, draped, anesthetized, and taken to the OR. The physician inserts the scope and visualizes some esophageal varices. The physician completes an injection sclerosis of the esophageal varices. What is the correct CPT code assigned?

Case 2

William Whitelock is brought to the OR today for evaluation of an anal lesion. The patient is prepped, draped, anesthetized, and taken to the OR. The physician uses a speculum to open up the anal cavity so that the lesion can be visualized. The physician then uses a laser to destroy the lesion and surrounding tissue to ensure the entire lesion was removed. What is the correct CPT code assigned?

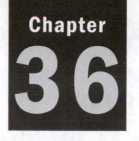
ENDOCRINE SYSTEM PROCEDURES

SCAVENGER HUNT

Go to the Justcoding website and Endocrine System coding quiz: http://www
.justcoding.com/quiz/2921

There are five questions to the quiz. How did you do on the quiz the first
try? How many times did it take you to get all five questions correct? What
are the correct answers for each of the five questions? Of the five questions,
which one was the hardest for you to find the correct code, and why?

APPLICATION ASSIGNMENT

Anatomy Labeling. Please identify the structures of the endocrine system
below by filling in the blanks:

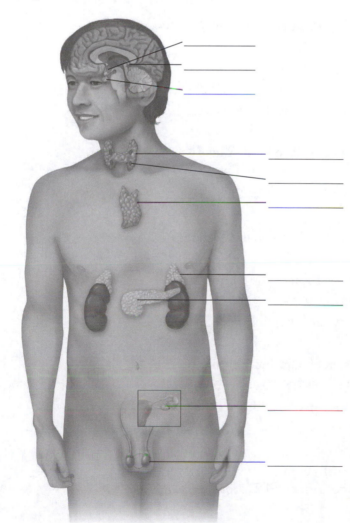

CRITICAL THINKING

Go to MedlinePlus, and watch the video on laparoscopic adrenalectomy via the following link: http://www.orlive.com/shawneemission/videos/laparoscopic-adrenalectomy1?view=displayPageNLM

After you watch the video, what was the most interesting part of it? As a coder, is it important to visually understand what you are coding? Why or why not? How do you think this video will be beneficial to you in your future coding career?

CODING CASES

1. Re-exploration of the parathyroid. What is the correct CPT code assigned?

2. Biopsy of the thyroid via a percutaneous core needle. What is the correct CPT code assigned?

3. Excision of carotid body tumor. What is the correct CPT code assigned?

4. I&D of infected thyroglossal duct cyst. What is the correct CPT code assigned?

5. Thyroidectomy with substernal thyroid. The procedure was completed via a cervical approach. What is the correct CPT code assigned?

6. Unlisted procedure, endocrine system. What is the correct CPT code assigned?

7. Subtotal thyroidectomy with limited neck dissection. What is the correct CPT code assigned?

8. Excision of adenoma of thyroid. What is the correct CPT code assigned?

9. Partial adrenalectomy with biopsy of the adrenal gland. What is the correct CPT code assigned?

10. Excision of carotid body tumor with excision of the carotid artery. What is the correct CPT code assigned?

11. Unilateral total thyroid lobectomy. What is the correct CPT code assigned?

12. Complete adrenalectomy with excision of adjacent retroperitoneal tumor. What is the correct CPT code assigned?

13. Excision of thyroglossal sinus. What is the correct CPT code assigned?

14. Excision of recurrent thyroglossal duct cyst. What is the correct CPT code assigned?

15. Partial unilateral thyroid lobectomy with contralateral subtotal lobectomy and isthmusectomy. What is the correct CPT code assigned?

16. Injection of a thyroid cyst. What is the correct CPT code assigned?

17. Complete thyroidectomy. What is the correct CPT code assigned?

18. Total unilateral thyroid lobectomy with isthmusectomy. What is the correct CPT code assigned?

19. Surgical laparoscopy with complete adrenalectomy. What is the correct CPT code assigned?

20. Transcervical total thymectomy. What is the correct CPT code assigned?

CODING PRACTICE

Case 1

Joseph Jamesson is seen today for treatment of thyroid cancer. The patient is taken to the OR, prepped, draped, and anesthetized. The surgeon completes a total thyroidectomy with radical neck dissection. What is the correct CPT code assigned?

Case 2

Beverly Benson is seen today for a parathyroidectomy. Beverly is taken to the OR, prepped, draped, and anesthetized. The surgeon completes a parathyroidectomy with mediastinal exploration, transthoracic approach with parathyroid autotransplantation. What is the correct CPT code assigned?

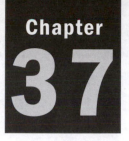

INTEGUMENTARY SYSTEM PROCEDURES

SCAVENGER HUNT

Go to the Justcoding website and Integumentary system coding quiz: http://www.justcoding.com/quiz/2660

There are five questions to the quiz. How did you do on the quiz the first try? How many times did it take you to get all five questions correct? What are the correct answers for each of the five questions? Of the five questions, which one was the hardest for you to find the correct code, and why?

APPLICATION ASSIGNMENT

Match the following skin signs with their definition:

_____ 1. Macule   a. a crack-like sore
_____ 2. Wheal   b. small, elevated skin lesion filled with pus
_____ 3. Papule   c. small fluid-filled sac
_____ 4. Pustule   d. a localized evanescent elevation of the skin
_____ 5. Erosion   e. an ulcer gnawing away tissue
_____ 6. Fissure   f. solid, elevated area on the skin
_____ 7. Vesicle   g. a discolored spot on the skin

CRITICAL THINKING

Go to MedlinePlus, and watch the video on breast reconstruction surgery via the following link: http://www.orlive.com/synovis-surgical-innovations/videos/breast-reconstruction-with-tissue-expansion/UPDATEAPP/false/VIEW/displayPageNLM

After you watch the video, what was the most interesting part of it? As a coder, is it important to visually understand what you are coding? Why or why not? How do you think this video will be beneficial to you in your future coding career?

CODING CASES

1. Intermediate repair of wound of the scalp. The repair was 6 cm in length. What is the correct CPT code assigned?

2. Dermal chemical facial peel. What is the correct CPT code assigned?

3. Complex repair of open wounds on the trunk. The wounds total 3 cm. What is the correct CPT code assigned?

4. Excision of trochanteric pressure ulcer with ostectomy. What is the correct CPT code assigned?

5. Blepharoplasty of the lower eyelid with an extensive herniated fat pad. What is the correct CPT code assigned?

6. Dressing change under anesthesia. What is the correct CPT code assigned?

7. Secondary closure of complicated wound dehiscence. What is the correct CPT code assigned?

8. Cryosurgery of malignant lesion of the leg that is 1.5 cm. What is the correct CPT code assigned?

9. Rhytidectomy of the forehead. What is the correct CPT code assigned?

10. Lumpectomy of the right breast. What is the correct CPT code assigned?

11. Adjacent tissue transfer of the forehead 5 cm. What is the correct CPT code assigned?

12. Debridement of partial-thickness burn to the thumb and index finger. What is the correct CPT code assigned?

13. Abrasion of 8 keratotic lesions. What is the correct CPT code assigned?

14. Bilateral breast reconstruction with free flap. What is the correct CPT code assigned?

15. Lipectomy of the buttocks. What is the correct CPT code assigned?

16. Dermal autograft of the left arm. What is the correct CPT code assigned?

17. Cryotherapy for acne. What is the correct CPT code assigned?

18. Cervicoplasty. What is the correct CPT code assigned?

19. Excision of a coccygeal pressure ulcer with coccygectomy and flap closure. What is the correct CPT code assigned?

20. Full-thickness free skin graft of the scalp that was 10 cm in length. What is the correct CPT code assigned?

CODING PRACTICE

Case 1

Thirty-seven-year-old Beverly Bronson is here for treatment of her right breast gynecomastia. Beverly is taken to the OR, prepped, draped, and anesthetized. The surgeon complete a mastectomy of her right breast without any complications. Patient is sent to recovery in stable condition. What is the correct CPT code assigned?

Case 2

Thomas Toon is brought to the OR for excision of a .8 cm basal cell carcinoma of his left nasal and nasolabial crease. He is taken to the OR, prepped, draped, and anesthetized. The specimen was removed with margins of .1 cm on both sides and sent to pathology. The wound was closed in layers using 4-0 Dexon to the deep tissues, and the skin was closed with #7-0 Ethilon interrupted simple fashion. What is the correct CPT code assigned?

MUSCULOSKELETAL SYSTEM PROCEDURES

SCAVENGER HUNT

Go to the Justcoding website and Musculoskeletal System coding quiz: http://www.justcoding.com/quiz/2969

There are five questions to the quiz. How did you do on the quiz the first try? How many times did it take you to get all five questions correct? What are the correct answers for each of the five questions? Of the five questions which one was the hardest for you to find the correct code, and why?

APPLICATION ASSIGNMENT

Anatomy Labeling. Please identify the structures of the musculoskeletal system by filling in the blanks:

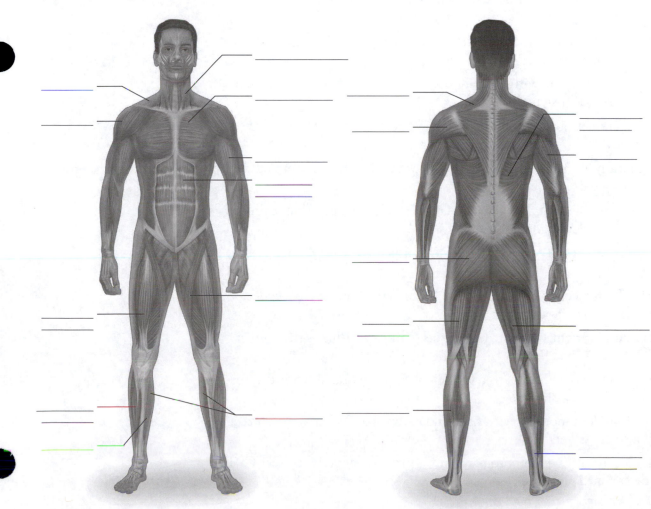

CRITICAL THINKING

Go to MedlinePlus, and watch the video on small incision total hip arthroplasty via the following link: http://www.orlive.com/mercyhospital/videos/two-procedures-small-incision-total-hip-arthroplasty?view=displaypageNLM

After you watch the video, what was the most interesting part of it? As a coder, is it important to visually understand what you are coding? Why or why not? How do you think this video will be beneficial to you in your future coding career?

CODING CASES

1. Radical resection of a sarcoma of the scalp that is 1.5 cm. What is the correct CPT code assigned?

2. Open treatment of a depressed zygomatic arch fracture. What is the correct CPT code assigned?

3. Biopsy of deep back tissue. What is the correct CPT code assigned?

4. Exploration of penetrating abdomen wound. What is the correct CPT code assigned?

5. Posterior arthrodesis for kyphosis, with cast for six vertebral segments. What is the correct CPT code assigned?

6. Osteotomy of spine with anterior discectomy C1-C2. What is the correct CPT code assigned?

7. Radical resection of a clavicle tumor. What is the correct CPT code assigned?

8. Aspiration of a ganglion cyst of the left wrist. What is the correct CPT code assigned?

9. Closed treatment of the proximal end of the left ulnar. What is the correct CPT code assigned?

10. Open treatment of a hyoid fracture. What is the correct CPT code assigned?

11. I&D of infected left shoulder bursa. What is the correct CPT code assigned?

12. Tenodesis at right wrist with extensors of fingers. What is the correct CPT code assigned?

13. Arthrocentesis with injection of the right knee bursa. What is the correct CPT code assigned?

14. Left shoulder tenotomy with one tendon repaired. What is the correct CPT code assigned?

15. Arthrotomy of the temporomandibular joint. What is the correct CPT code assigned?

16. Open treatment of a thoracic vertebral fracture, posterior approach. What is the correct CPT code assigned?

17. Arthrodesis, anterior interbody technique with discectomy T5-T6. What is the correct CPT code assigned?

18. Impression and custom preparation of an orbital prosthesis. What is the correct CPT code assigned?

19. Closed treatment of a nasal septal fracture. What is the correct CPT code assigned?

20. Invasive electrical stimulation to aid bone healing. What is the correct CPT code assigned?

CODING PRACTICE

Case 1

Christopher Chumb is being seen today for replantation of his right thumb following an MVA in which there was a complete amputation. Christopher was taken to the OR, prepped, draped, and given a block. The surgeon completed an amputation from the distal tip to the MIP joint of Christopher's right hand. What is the correct CPT code assigned?

Case 2

Raymond Reclick is here for a Krukenberg procedure. Raymond is taken to the OR, prepped, draped, and placed in the supine position. Anesthesia is given. The surgeon completes an outline of where the amputation will be completed. The incision is then started and a Krukenberg procedure is successfully completed. The patient is taken to recovery in stable condition. What is the correct CPT code assigned?

CARDIOVASCULAR SYSTEM PROCEDURES

⬤ SCAVENGER HUNT

Go to the Justcoding website and Cardiovascular System procedures coding quiz: http://www.justcoding.com/quiz/2791

There are five questions to the quiz. How did you do on the quiz the first try? How many times did it take you to get all five questions correct? What are the correct answers for each of the five questions? Of the five questions, which one was the hardest for you to find the correct code, and why?

⬤ APPLICATION ASSIGNMENT

Anatomy Labeling. Please identify the structures of the cardiovascular system by filling in the blanks:

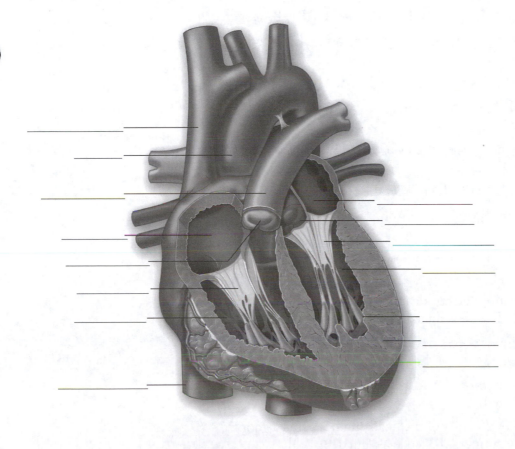

CRITICAL THINKING

Go to MedlinePlus, and watch the video on Coronary Angioplasty via the following link: http://www.orlive.com/shawneemission/videos/coronary-angioplasty-stent-placement?view=displayPageNLM

After you watch the video, what was the most interesting part of it? As a coder, is it important to visually understand what you are coding? Why or why not? How do you think this video will be beneficial to you in your future coding career?

CODING CASES

1. Replacement of the pulmonary valve. What is the correct CPT code assigned?

2. Pulmonary artery embolectomy. What is the correct CPT code assigned?

3. Endovascular repair of iliac artery. What is the correct CPT code assigned?

4. Closure of AV valve by suture. What is the correct CPT code assigned?

5. Therapeutic apheresis for platelets. What is the correct CPT code assigned?

6. Donor cardiectomy. What is the correct CPT code assigned?

7. Repair of tetralogy of Fallot with transannular patch. What is the correct CPT code assigned?

8. Collection of capillary blood specimen via ear stick. What is the correct CPT code assigned?

9. Tube pericardiostomy. What is the correct CPT code assigned?

10. Ligation of the common carotid artery. What is the correct CPT code assigned?

11. Right radial thrombectomy by incision. What is the correct CPT code assigned?

12. Repair of single transvenous electrode in implantable defibrillator. What is the correct CPT code assigned?

13. Insertion of central venous access device in a 2-year-old. What is the correct CPT code assigned?

14. Percutaneous insertion of intra-aortic balloon assist device. What is the correct CPT code assigned?

15. Repair of a congenital AV fistula of the head and neck in a 2-month-old infant. What is the correct CPT code assigned?

16. Newborn umbilical artery catheterization. What is the correct CPT code assigned?

17. Left leg valvuloplasty of the femoral vein. What is the correct CPT code assigned?

18. Removal of permanent pacemaker pulse generator only. What is the correct CPT code assigned?

19. Division of aberrant vessel with reanastomosis. What is the correct CPT code assigned?

20. CABG, 2 coronary venous grafts. What is the correct CPT code assigned?

CODING PRACTICE

Case 1

Sally Simrod is a 44-year-old patient with breast carcinoma of the left breast. Sally is brought into the OR today for placement of a central venous access device so that she can start chemotherapy. Sally is prepped, draped, anesthetized, and taken to the OR. The physician makes an incision over the subclavian area and places a central venous catheter at the subclavian vein. The catheter is checked and is working properly. The patient will start chemotherapy the following day and is discharged to follow up the next morning for chemotherapy. What is the correct CPT code assigned?

Case 2

Patty Paddington was seen earlier today for severe swelling and redness, which is hot to touch, in her lower extremities. It was determined that Patty has a thrombus in her popliteal area, so she will be taken to surgery to remove this. After the initial review, the physician makes an incision over the popliteal-tibio-peroneal artery and removes small thrombi successfully without any complications. Patient is sent to recovery in stable condition. What is the correct CPT code assigned?

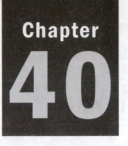

HEMIC AND LYMPHATIC SYSTEMS, MEDIASTINUM, AND DIAPHRAGM PROCEDURES

SCAVENGER HUNT

Go to the Justcoding website and mediastinum coding quiz: http://www.justcoding.com/quiz/2885

There are five questions to the quiz. How did you do on the quiz the first try? How many times did it take you to get all five questions correct? What are the correct answers for each of the five questions? Of the five questions, which one was the hardest for you to find the correct code, and why?

APPLICATION ASSIGNMENT

Anatomy Labeling. Please identify the structures of the lymphatic system by filling in the blanks:

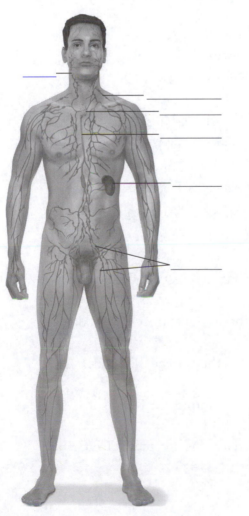

CRITICAL THINKING

Go to MedlinePlus, and watch the video on a tonsillectomy via the following link: http://www.orlive.com/arthrocare-corporation/videos/coblation-an-advanced-pediatric-tonsillectomy?view=displayPageNLM

After you watch the video, what was the most interesting part of it? As a coder, is it important to visually understand what you are coding? Why or why not? How do you think this video will be beneficial to you in your future coding career?

CODING CASES

1. Aspiration of bone marrow. What is the correct CPT code assigned?

2. Resection of mediastinal cyst. What is the correct CPT code assigned?

3. Total splenectomy. What is the correct CPT code assigned?

4. Modified radical neck dissection. What is the correct CPT code assigned?

5. Laparoscopy with bilateral total pelvic lymphadenectomy. What is the correct CPT code assigned?

6. Pelvic lymphadenectomy with external iliac, hypogastric, and obturator nodes. What is the correct CPT code assigned?

7. Repair a laceration of the diaphragm. What is the correct CPT code assigned?

8. Mediastinoscopy with biopsy. What is the correct CPT code assigned?

9. Injection procedure for a bilateral lymphangiography. What is the correct CPT code assigned?

10. Laparoscopic splenectomy. What is the correct CPT code assigned?

11. Thoracic duct cannulation. What is the correct CPT code assigned?

12. Needle biopsy of axillary lymph nodes. What is the correct CPT code assigned?

13. Simple drainage of lymphadenitis. What is the correct CPT code assigned?

14. Removal of a 3 cm mediastinal tumor. What is the correct CPT code assigned?

15. Deep cervical lymph node excision. What is the correct CPT code assigned?

16. Dissection of deep jugular nodes. What is the correct CPT code assigned?

17. Bilateral suprahyoid lympadenectomy. What is the correct CPT code assigned?

18. Transplant preparation of hematopoietic progenitor cells; thawing of previously frozen harvest with washing. What is the correct CPT code assigned?

19. Repair of newborn diaphragmatic hernia. What is the correct CPT code assigned?

20. Allogeneic bone marrow harvesting for transplant. What is the correct CPT code assigned?

CODING PRACTICE

Case 1

Forty-five-year-old Isabelle Islet was involved in an MVA when the car she was driving collided with a deer. She was taken by ambulance to the ER, where an emergency splenorrhaphy was performed. What is the correct CPT code assigned?

Case 2

Twenty-eight-year-old Billy Baker was brought to the OR for an excision of a cervical cystic hygroma. The patient was prepped, draped, and placed in the supine position. Spinal anesthesia was administered and an excision was made over the cervical region. The physician removed the cystic hygroma with deep neurovascular dissection as well. What is the correct CPT code assigned?

RESPIRATORY SYSTEM PROCEDURES

SCAVENGER HUNT

Go to the Justcoding website and Respiratory System coding quiz: http://www .justcoding.com/quiz/2885

There are five questions to the quiz. How did you do on the quiz the first try? How many times did it take you to get all five questions correct? What are the correct answers for each of the five questions? Of the five questions, which one was the hardest for you to find the correct code, and why?

APPLICATION ASSIGNMENT

Anatomy Labeling. Please identify the structures of the respiratory system by filling in the blanks:

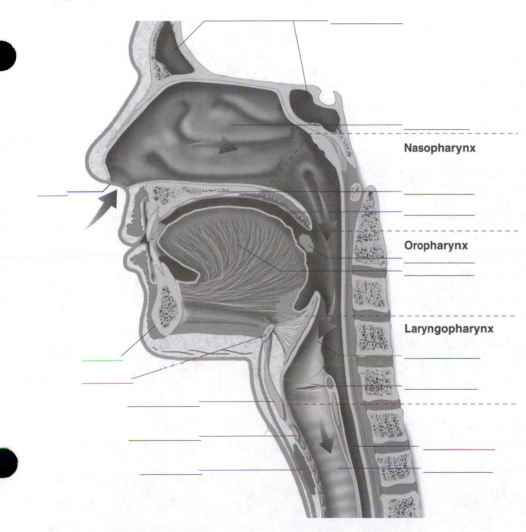

CRITICAL THINKING

Go to MedlinePlus, and watch the video on lung cancer via the following link: http://www.orlive.com/chp/videos/minimally-invasive-treatment-for-lung-cancer?view=displayPageNLM

After you watch the video what was the most interesting part of it? As a coder, is it important to visually understand what you are coding? Why or why not? How do you think this video will be beneficial to you in your future coding career?

CODING CASES

1. Schede thoracoplasty with closure of bronchopleural fistula. What is the correct CPT code assigned?

2. Thoracoscopy with biopsy of pleura. What is the correct CPT code assigned?

3. Completion pneumonectomy. What is the correct CPT code assigned?

4. Pleurodesis with instillation of talc. What is the correct CPT code assigned?

5. Removal of tunneled indwelling pleural catheter with cuff. What is the correct CPT code assigned?

6. Carinal reconstruction. What is the correct CPT code assigned?

7. Total lung lavage. What is the correct CPT code assigned?

8. Emergency ET intubation in the ER. What is the correct CPT code assigned?

9. Flexible bronchoscopy with fluoroscopic guidance and bronchial alveolar lavage. What is the correct CPT code assigned?

10. Thoracentesis with imaging guidance via catheter with aspiration of the pleural cavity. What is the correct CPT code assigned?

11. Therapeutic pneumothorax with intrapleural injection of air. What is the correct CPT code assigned?

12. Anterior nasal package for recurrent bilateral epistaxis. What is the correct CPT code assigned?

13. Sinus endoscopy with sphenoidotomy. What is the correct CPT code assigned?

14. Bilateral excision of nasal polyps. What is the correct CPT code assigned?

15. Thoracoscopy with segmentectomy. What is the correct CPT code assigned?

16. Extrapleural removal of lung. What is the correct CPT code assigned?

17. Laryngectomy with radical neck dissection. What is the correct CPT code assigned?

18. Empyemectomy. What is the correct CPT code assigned?

19. Direct laryngoscopy with infection into the vocal cords. What is the correct CPT code assigned?

20. Thoracoscopy with lobectomy. What is the correct CPT code assigned?

CODING PRACTICE

Case 1

Forty-four-year-old Margaret Miler has had severe, recurrent sinusitis for years. She has tried traditional methods and nothing is working to relieve her symptoms. She is taken to surgery for a maxillary sinusotomy. The patient is prepped, draped, and anesthetized. The surgeon makes an incision and visualizes the maxillary sinus. He notes antrochoanal polyps and removes these via forceps. The remaining procedure is completed without any complications. What is the correct CPT code assigned?

Case 2

Thirty-seven-year-old Matthew Manger is admitted for an exploration of his sinuses. Matthew is taken to the OR, where is he prepped, draped, and anesthetized. The physician inserts the scope and enters the frontal sinus and removes some tissue. The tissue is sent to pathology. What is the correct CPT code assigned?

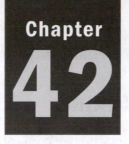

NERVOUS SYSTEM PROCEDURES

SCAVENGER HUNT

Go to the Justcoding website and Nervous System procedures coding quiz:
http://www.justcoding.com/quiz/2815

There are five questions to the quiz. How did you do on the quiz the first
try? How many times did it take you to get all five questions correct? What
are the correct answers for each of the five questions? Of the five questions,
which one was the hardest for you to find the correct code, and why?

APPLICATION ASSIGNMENT

Anatomy Labeling. Please identify the structures of the nervous system by
filling in the blanks:

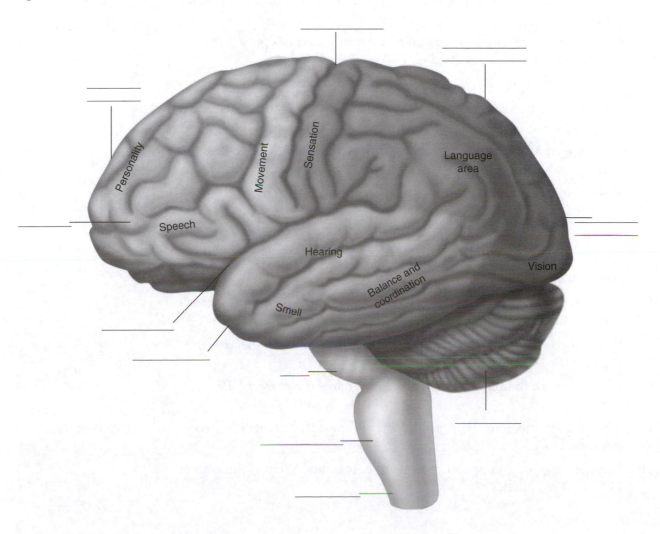

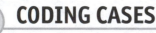

CRITICAL THINKING

Go to MedlinePlus, and watch the video on carpal tunnel surgery via the following link: http://www.orlive.com/hartfordhospital/videos/carpal-tunnel-release?view=displayPageNLM

After you watch the video, what was the most interesting part of it? As a coder, is it important to visually understand what you are coding? Why or why not? How do you think this video will be beneficial to you in your future coding career?

CODING CASES

1. Cranial decompression of the posterior fossa. What is the correct CPT code assigned?

2. Ventriculocisternostomy. What is the correct CPT code assigned?

3. Craniectomy for implantation of cortical, cerebellar neurostimulator electrodes. What is the correct CPT code assigned?

4. Reprogramming of cerebrospinal shunt. What is the correct CPT code assigned?

5. Laminectomy with decompression of the spinal cord L3-L4. What is the correct CPT code assigned?

6. Cisternal puncture. What is the correct CPT code assigned?

7. Percutaneous needle biopsy of the spinal cord. What is the correct CPT code assigned?

8. Irrigation of subarachnoid catheter. What is the correct CPT code assigned?

9. A 4-cm meningocele repaired without complications. What is the correct CPT code assigned?

10. Craniectomy for osteomyelitis. What is the correct CPT code assigned?

11. Injection of anesthetic into the vagus nerve. What is the correct CPT code assigned?

12. Craniotomy with repair of an encephalocele at the skull base. What is the correct CPT code assigned?

13. Percutaneous implant of a neuromuscular neurostimulator electrode. What is the correct CPT code assigned?

14. Burr hole with drainage of brain abscess. What is the correct CPT code assigned?

15. Thoracic laminectomy with myelotomy. What is the correct CPT code assigned?

16. Craniectomy for evacuation of subdural hematoma. What is the correct CPT code assigned?

17. Laminotomy with decompression of nerve roots and excision of herniated intervertebral disc, C5-C6. What is the correct CPT code assigned?

18. Diagnostic lumbar puncture. What is the correct CPT code assigned?

19. Repair of a simple dural AV malformation. What is the correct CPT code assigned?

20. Craniotomy with elevation of bone flap for temporal lobectomy. What is the correct CPT code assigned?

CODING PRACTICE

Case 1

Sixteen-year-old Emma Ellison was involved in an MVA when her car rolled over and she was ejected. Emma has a piece of metal that is lodged into her skull, and she is immediately taken to surgery. The neurosurgeon performed a craniectomy with excision of the metal and closure of the penetrating open wound of the brain. Emma is sent to ICU for recovery. What is the correct CPT code assigned?

Case 2

Eight-year-old Gavin Georgeson has recurrent chronic seizures. He is brought to surgery today to have electrodes implanted to monitor his seizures. He is taken to surgery, where he is prepped, draped, and anesthetized. The surgeon performs a stereotactic implantation of depth electrodes into the cerebrum. What is the correct CPT code assigned?

EYE AND OCULAR ADNEXA PROCEDURES

SCAVENGER HUNT

Go to the Justcoding website and Eye coding quiz: http://www.justcoding .com/quiz/2847

There are five questions to the quiz. How did you do on the quiz the first try? How many times did it take you to get all five questions correct? What are the correct answers for each of the five questions? Of the five questions, which one was the hardest for you to find the correct code, and why?

APPLICATION ASSIGNMENT

Anatomy Labeling. Please identify the structures of the eye by filling in the blanks:

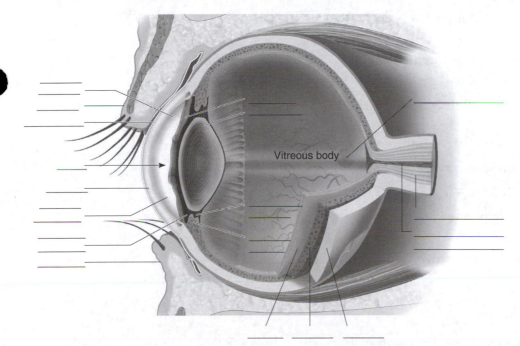

Vitreous body

CRITICAL THINKING

Go to MedlinePlus, and watch the video on diabetic vitrectomy via the following link: http://www.orlive.com/shawneemission/videos/ diabetic-vitrectomy-surgery?view=displayPageNLM

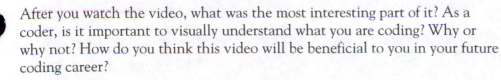

After you watch the video, what was the most interesting part of it? As a coder, is it important to visually understand what you are coding? Why or why not? How do you think this video will be beneficial to you in your future coding career?

CODING CASES

1. Removal of intraocular foreign body from the anterior chamber of the right eye. What is the correct CPT code assigned?

2. Intracapsular removal of lens material via aspiration on the right eye. What is the correct CPT code assigned?

3. Strabismus surgery of the superior oblique muscle in the right eye. What is the correct CPT code assigned?

4. Enucleation of left eye. What is the correct CPT code assigned?

5. ICCE with insertion of intraocular lens prosthesis of the right eye. What is the correct CPT code assigned?

6. Excision of sclera lesion. What is the correct CPT code assigned?

7. Bilateral canthotomy. What is the correct CPT code assigned?

8. Subconjunctival injection. What is the correct CPT code assigned?

9. Biopsy of cornea of the left eye. What is the correct CPT code assigned?

10. I&D of the right lacrimal gland. What is the correct CPT code assigned?

11. Removal of blood clot from the anterior segment of the right eye. What is the correct CPT code assigned?

12. Scleral reinforcement with graft. What is the correct CPT code assigned?

13. Bilateral repair of canaliculi. What is the correct CPT code assigned?

14. Epikeratoplasty. What is the correct CPT code assigned?

15. Exchange of intraocular lens. What is the correct CPT code assigned?

16. Extraocular removal of implanted material from the posterior segment of the left eye. What is the correct CPT code assigned?

17. Diagnostic scraping of the left cornea. What is the correct CPT code assigned?

18. Thermaocauterization of ectroprion. What is the correct CPT code assigned?

19. Repair of right scleral staphyloma with graft. What is the correct CPT code assigned?

20. Radical keratotomy. What is the correct CPT code assigned?

CODING PRACTICE

Case 1

Allison Avery is an 18-month-old who has had repeated conjunctivitis due to clogged lacrimal ducts. She is brought to surgery today to have these probed. Allison is prepped, draped, and anesthetized. She is taken to the OR suite, and the physician probes her right lacrimal duct and irrigates this. He then completes the same procedure on the left side. Allison is taken to recovery and sent home with her parents. What is the correct CPT code assigned?

Case 2

Magdolio McCleain is a 77-year-old seen today for senile cataracts. Magdolio has these in both eyes, but the right is more severe than the left. She is prepped, draped, given anesthesia, and taken to the OR. The physician performs a complete ECCE with insertion of intraocular lens prosthesis of the right eye. Magdolio is taken to recovery in stable condition and will follow up with the ophthalmologist in 2 weeks. What is the correct CPT code assigned?

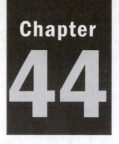
AUDITORY SYSTEM PROCEDURES AND OPERATING MICROSCOPE PROCEDURES

SCAVENGER HUNT

Go to the Justcoding website and auditory system procedures coding quiz:
http://www.justcoding.com/quiz/2766

There are five questions to the quiz. How did you do on the quiz the first try? How many times did it take you to get all five questions correct? What are the correct answers for each of the five questions? Of the five questions, which one was the hardest for you to find the correct code, and why?

APPLICATION ASSIGNMENT

Anatomy Labeling. Please identify the structures of the ear by filling in the blanks:

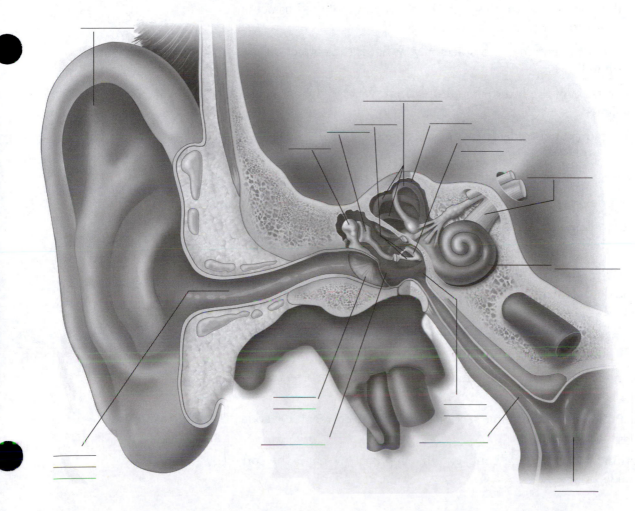

CRITICAL THINKING

Go to MedlinePlus, and watch the video on myringotomy via the following link: http://orlive.com/broward-health/videos/bilateral-myringotomy-tube-placement?view=displayPageNLM

After you watch the video, what was the most interesting part of it? As a coder, is it important to visually understand what you are coding? Why or why not? How do you think this video will be beneficial to you in your future coding career?

CODING CASES

1. Bilateral decompression of the internal auditory canal. What is the correct CPT code assigned?

2. Excision of an aural polyp in the left ear. What is the correct CPT code assigned?

3. Transcanal labyrinthectomy with mastoidectomy. What is the correct CPT code assigned?

4. Bilateral myringotomy with aspiration and inflation of the Eustachian tube. What is the correct CPT code assigned?

5. Revision mastoidectomy with apicetomy. What is the correct CPT code assigned?

6. Decompression of the internal auditory canal. What is the correct CPT code assigned?

7. Modified radical mastoidectomy. What is the correct CPT code assigned?

8. Transcanal tympanolysis. What is the correct CPT code assigned?

9. Cochlear device implantation. What is the correct CPT code assigned?

10. Otoplasty of the left ear for a protruding ear. What is the correct CPT code assigned?

11. Bilateral myringoplasty. What is the correct CPT code assigned?

12. Routine debridement of the right mastoidectomy cavity. What is the correct CPT code assigned?

13. Endolymphatic sac operation with shunt. What is the correct CPT code assigned?

14. Excision of transcanal aural glomus tumor. What is the correct CPT code assigned?

15. Transcranial vestibular nerve section. What is the correct CPT code assigned?

16. Resection of the temporal bone, external approach. What is the correct CPT code assigned?

17. Complicated drainage of an external hematoma of the left ear. What is the correct CPT code assigned?

18. Revision of stapedectomy. What is the correct CPT code assigned?

19. Left ear repair round window fistula. What is the correct CPT code assigned?

20. Fenestration of the semicircular canal of the right ear. What is the correct CPT code assigned?

CODING PRACTICE

Case 1

Fifty-five-year-old Joseph Jones is a farmer who has been having difficulty hearing. On examination, it is determined that Joseph has severe cerumen impaction. Joseph is taken to the SDS suite, prepped, draped, and given anesthesia. The physician uses the instrument to clean out both ear canals and removes copious amounts of dirty cerumen. The patient is allowed to wake up and is transferred to recovery and discharged home to follow up as needed. What is the correct CPT code assigned?

Case 2

Eight-year-old Nicholas Nicols has had recurrent otitis media that is chronic and unresponsive to medication. Nicholas was brought to the SDS suite, prepped, draped, and given anesthesia. A bilateral tympanoplasty with mastoidectomy is performed on both ears without complication. Nicholas is discharged home and will follow up in 2 weeks. What is the correct CPT code assigned?

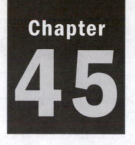

URINARY AND MALE GENITAL SYSTEM PROCEDURES

SCAVENGER HUNT

Go to the Justcoding website and Urinary System coding quiz: http://www
.justcoding.com/quiz/2924

There are five questions to the quiz. How did you do on the quiz the first
try? How many times did it take you to get all five questions correct? What
are the correct answers for each of the five questions? Of the five questions,
which one was the hardest for you to find the correct code, and why?

APPLICATION ASSIGNMENT

Anatomy Labeling. Please identify the structures of the urinary system by
filling in the blanks:

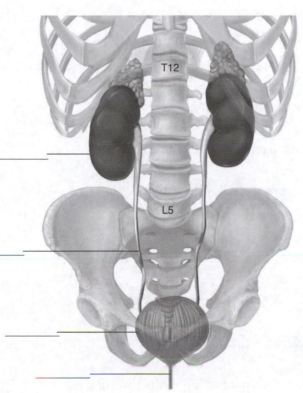

CRITICAL THINKING

Go to MedlinePlus, and watch the video on a circumcision via the following
link: http://peds.broadcastmed.com/4229/videos/circumcision?view=display
PageNLM

After you watch the video, what was the most interesting part of it? As a coder, is it important to visually understand what you are coding? Why or why not? How do you think this video will be beneficial to you in your future coding career?

CODING CASES

1. Excision of perinephric cyst. What is the correct CPT code assigned?

2. Nephrotomy with exploration. What is the correct CPT code assigned?

3. Ureterotomy for insertion of indwelling stent. What is the correct CPT code assigned?

4. Needle aspiration of bladder. What is the correct CPT code assigned?

5. Pyelotomy with exploration. What is the correct CPT code assigned?

6. Cutaneous vesicostomy. What is the correct CPT code assigned?

7. Complete cystectomy. What is the correct CPT code assigned?

8. Partial nephrectomy of the right kidney. What is the correct CPT code assigned?

9. Utereroureterostomy. What is the correct CPT code assigned?

10. Nephrolithotomy with removal of calculus. What is the correct CPT code assigned?

11. EMG of the urethral sphincter. What is the correct CPT code assigned?

12. Needle biopsy of the left kidney. What is the correct CPT code assigned?

13. Bladder installation of anticarcinogenic agent. What is the correct CPT code assigned?

14. Complex uroflowmetry. What is the correct CPT code assigned?

15. Ureteroplasty for ureteral stricture. What is the correct CPT code assigned?

16. Removal of transplanted renal allograft. What is the correct CPT code assigned?

17. Extracorporeal shock wave lithotripsy. What is the correct CPT code assigned?

18. Closure of ureterocutaneous fistula. What is the correct CPT code assigned?

19. Percutaneous removal and replacement via snare of internally dwelling left stent with radiological supervision and interpretation. What is the correct CPT code assigned?

20. Percutaneous nephrostolithotomy with basket extraction. What is the correct CPT code assigned?

CODING PRACTICE

Case 1

Fifty-four-year-old Helen Hall is seen today for treatment of her stress incontinence. Helen was prepped, draped, anesthetized, and taken to the OR. A laparoscope was inserted where a urethral suspension was completed without any complications. Helen was transferred to the recovery room and discharged home to follow up in 2 weeks. What is the correct CPT code assigned?

Case 2

Benjamin Betty was diagnosed with carcinoma of the bladder last month after a CT scan showed a 4-cm tumor in the neck of the bladder. Today Benjamin is brought to the OR for a cystourethroscopy with resection of the tumor. The patient is prepped, draped, and given anesthesia. The physician inserts the scope and visualizes the tumor. He removes the tumor and margins and sends it to pathology for review. The patient is transferred to the recovery room in stable condition. What is the correct CPT code assigned?

FEMALE GENITAL SYSTEM, MATERNITY CARE, AND DELIVERY PROCEDURES

SCAVENGER HUNT

Go to the Justcoding website and Maternity Care coding quiz: http://www.justcoding.com/quiz/2842

There are five questions to the quiz. How did you do on the quiz the first try? How many times did it take you to get all five questions correct? What are the correct answers for each of the five questions? Of the five questions, which one was the hardest for you to find the correct code, and why?

APPLICATION ASSIGNMENT

Anatomy Labeling. Please identify the structures of the female reproductive system by filling in the blanks:

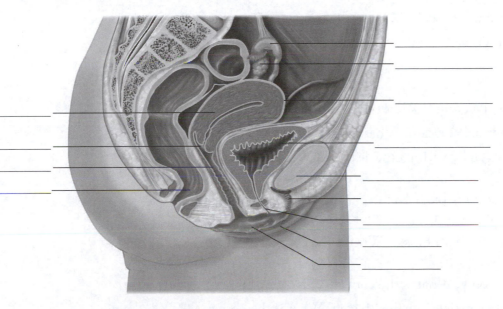

CRITICAL THINKING

Go to MedlinePlus, and watch the video on a C-section via the following link: http://www.orlive.com/shawneemission/videos/cesarean-section-birth?view=displayPageNLM

After you watch the video, what was the most interesting part of it? As a coder, is it important to visually understand what you are coding? Why or why not? How do you think this video will be beneficial to you in your future coding career?

CODING CASES

1. Lysis of labial adhesions. What is the correct CPT code assigned?

2. Irrigation of vagina with fungal medication. What is the correct CPT code assigned?

3. Colpocentesis. What is the correct CPT code assigned?

4. Abdominal excision of cervical stump with pelvic floor repair. What is the correct CPT code assigned?

5. Wedge resection of right ovary. What is the correct CPT code assigned?

6. Incision and drainage of Bartholin's gland abscess. What is the correct CPT code assigned?

7. Sling operation for stress incontinence. What is the correct CPT code assigned?

8. Plastic repair of a urethrocele. What is the correct CPT code assigned?

9. Endocervical curettage. What is the correct CPT code assigned?

10. Vaginal repair of an enterocele. What is the correct CPT code assigned?

11. Partial radical vulvectomy. What is the correct CPT code assigned?

12. Endometrial thermal ablation. What is the correct CPT code assigned?

13. Posterior colporrhaphy with rectocele repair. What is the correct CPT code assigned?

14. Supracervical laparoscopic hysterectomy with bilateral salpingo-oophorectomy. What is the correct CPT code assigned?

15. Colposcopy of vulva with biopsy. What is the correct CPT code assigned?

16. Partial hymenectomy. What is the correct CPT code assigned?

17. Construction of artificial vagina with graft. What is the correct CPT code assigned?

18. LeFort procedure on the vagina. What is the correct CPT code assigned?

19. Vaginectomy with removal of paravaginal tissue. What is the correct CPT code assigned?

20. Biopsy of two vulva lesions. What is the correct CPT code assigned?

CODING PRACTICE

Case 1

Sophia Swenson is a 25-year-old female gravida 1 para 0 seen today for a stress test. Patient is brought in and hooked up to the fetal monitor. A fetal contraction stress test was performed without any complications. The stress test looked good, and she is to follow up in 1 week. What is the correct CPT code assigned?

Case 2

Twenty-year-old Hannah Hart is seen today for persistent vaginal condyloma. She is prepped, draped, and given local anesthesia. The physician then completes extensive laser surgery to destroy the multiple vaginal condyloma present. What is the correct CPT code assigned?

RADIOLOGY SERVICES

SCAVENGER HUNT

Go to the Justcoding website and Radiology coding quiz: http://www .justcoding.com/quiz/2946

There are five questions to the quiz. How did you do on the quiz the first try? How many times did it take you to get all five questions correct? What are the correct answers for each of the five questions? Of the five questions, which one was the hardest for you to find the correct code, and why?

APPLICATION ASSIGNMENT

Match the correct positional term with the correct definition

_____ 1. Supine Position	a. the patient is placed with the front part of the body facing the x-ray tube and the back of the body facing the film.
_____ 2. Lateral Position	
_____ 3. Oblique Position (Lat)	b. the patient is placed with the back part of the body facing the x-ray tube and the front of the body facing the film.
_____ 4. Prone Position	
_____ 5. Anteroposterior Position (AP)	c. the x-ray beam passes from one side of the patient's body to the opposite side to reach the film.
_____ 6. Posteroanterior Position (PA)	

a. the patient is placed with the front part of the body facing the x-ray tube and the back of the body facing the film.

b. the patient is placed with the back part of the body facing the x-ray tube and the front of the body facing the film.

c. the x-ray beam passes from one side of the patient's body to the opposite side to reach the film.

d. the patient rests on the back, face upward, allowing the x-rays to pass through the body from the front to the back

e. the patient is placed lying facedown with the head turned to one side.

f. the patient is placed so that the body or body part to be imaged is at an angle to the x-ray beam

CRITICAL THINKING

Go to MedlinePlus, and watch the video on a transesophageal echocardiogram via the following link: http://www.orlive.com/shawneemission/videos/transesophageal-echocardiogram-tee-?view=displayPageNLM

After you watch the video, what was the most interesting part of it? As a coder, is it important to visually understand what you are coding? Why or why not? How do you think this video will be beneficial to you in your future coding career?

CODING CASES

1. Lumbosacral myelography with radiological supervision and interpretation. What is the correct CPT code assigned?

2. CT of the maxillofacial area with contrast material. What is the correct CPT code assigned?

3. Hypotonic duodenography. What is the correct CPT code assigned?

4. Bilateral pelvic lymphangiography with supervision and interpretation. What is the correct CPT code assigned?

5. CT of the lumbar spine with contrast material. What is the correct CPT code assigned?

6. Orthodontic cephalogram. What is the correct CPT code assigned?

7. Bilateral extremity angiography with supervision and interpretation. What is the correct CPT code assigned?

8. Two-view radiologic examination of the great toe. What is the correct CPT code assigned?

9. A-scan ophthalmic biometry ultrasound echography. What is the correct CPT code assigned?

10. Peringeogram. What is the correct CPT code assigned?

11. Magnetic resonance angiography of the head without contrast. What is the correct CPT code assigned?

12. Chest ultrasound with real-time image documentation. What is the correct CPT code assigned?

13. Complete hip radiologic examination. What is the correct CPT code assigned?

14. Transrectal ultrasound. What is the correct CPT code assigned?

15. Unilateral radiologic examination of the ribs, two views. What is the correct CPT code assigned?

16. Cardiac MRI for morphology and function with velocity flow mapping. What is the correct CPT code assigned?

17. Cervical discography with radiologic supervision and interpretation. What is the correct CPT code assigned?

18. Hepatic free venography with hemodynamic evaluation and supervision and interpretation. What is the correct CPT code assigned?

19. Videoradiography swallowing function. What is the correct CPT code assigned?

20. CT of the thorax. What is the correct CPT code assigned?

CODING PRACTICE

Case 1

Sally Stetson is a 47-year-old female with a family history of breast cancer. Both her maternal grandmother and sister have had breast cancer by the age of 50. Sally presents today for a screening mammogram. A bilateral screening mammogram with a two-view film from each breast was completed without any complications. What is the correct CPT code assigned?

Case 2

Casey Crimson is a 65-year-old male with non-small-cell lung carcinoma of his right lung. Casey has completed a chemotherapy treatment, and his cancer responded well to the chemotherapy, but the physician feels that they can still shrink the cancer even more with radiation. Casey presents today for a radiation treatment planning with Dr. Oscar, who will be the oncologist overseeing his radiation. Dr. Oscar performs an intermediate therapeutic radiation treatment plan with Casey. The treatments will begin on Monday and will be every weekday for 7 weeks. What is the correct CPT code assigned?

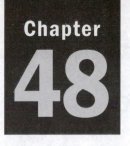

PATHOLOGY AND LABORATORY SERVICES

SCAVENGER HUNT

Go to the Justcoding website and Pathology and Laboratory coding quiz:
http://www.justcoding.com/quiz/2599

There are five questions to the quiz. How did you do on the quiz the first
try? How many times did it take you to get all five questions correct? What
are the correct answers for each of the five questions? Of the five questions,
which one was the hardest for you to find the correct code, and why?

APPLICATION ASSIGNMENT

Match the following characteristics of tumors to benign or malignant

_____	1. Grow slowly	a.	benign or malignant
_____	2. Grow rapidly	b.	benign or malignant
_____	3. Encapsulated	c.	benign or malignant
_____	4. Not encapsulated	d.	benign or malignant
_____	5. Cells resemble normal cells	e.	benign or malignant
_____	6. Cells undergo permanent change	f.	benign or malignant
_____	7. Remain localized	g.	benign or malignant
_____	8. Spread via the bloodstream	h.	benign or malignant

CRITICAL THINKING

Go to MedlinePlus, and watch the video on an ovarian mass via
the following link: http://onc.broadcastmed.com/3925/videos/
scarless-hysterectomy?view=displayPageNLM

After you watch the video, what was the most interesting part of it? As a
coder, is it important to visually understand what you are coding? Why or
why not? How do you think this video will be beneficial to you in your future
coding career?

CODING CASES

1. Therapeutic drug assay for caffeine. What is the correct CPT Code assigned?

2. Screening for chlorinated hydrocarbons. What is the correct CPT Code assigned?

3. Blood gases, pH only. What is the correct CPT Code assigned?

4. Surgical pathology for a vein varicosity. What is the correct CPT Code assigned?

5. Aldosterone suppression evaluation panel. What is the correct CPT Code assigned?

6. Sweat collection by iontophoresis. What is the correct CPT Code assigned?

7. Dexamethasone suppression test. What is the correct CPT Code assigned?

8. Total insulin. What is the correct CPT Code assigned?

9. Comprehensive pathology consultation with review of the patient's history and past medical records. What is the correct CPT Code assigned?

10. Surgical pathology for a missed abortion. What is the correct CPT Code assigned?

11. Bone marrow, smear, interpretation. What is the correct CPT Code assigned?

12. Surgical pathology for a left lung lobe resection. What is the correct CPT Code assigned?

13. Quantitative allergen specific IgE. What is the correct CPT Code assigned?

14. Qualitative urinalysis. What is the correct CPT Code assigned?

15. Oocyte identification from follicular fluid. What is the correct CPT Code assigned?

16. Free hydroxyproline. What is the correct CPT Code assigned?

17. Surgical pathology for simple breast mastectomy. What is the correct CPT Code assigned?

18. Qualitative ketone bodies. What is the correct CPT Code assigned?

19. Reticulated platelet assay. What is the correct CPT Code assigned?

20. Alpha-fetoprotein serum. What is the correct CPT Code assigned?

CODING PRACTICE

Case 1

Sixty-five-year-old William White has been having urinary retention and nocturia. He was examined by Dr. Smith, a urologist, who determined that William is suffering from hypertrophy of the prostate and scheduled a TURP. William was prepped, draped, and anesthetized. He was taken to the OR, where the scope was inserted and a resection of the enlarged prostate was removed without difficulty. The prostatic tissue was sent to pathology for review. What is the correct pathology CPT Code assigned?

Case 2

Twenty-two-year-old Zoey Zerber is seen today in the office for her routine annual wellness visit. Dr. Joseph completed a complete history and physical, examination and orders a general health panel to test her CBC, differential WBC, and TSH. He also orders a lipid panel to get a baseline cholesterol reading on Zoey. What is the correct CPT laboratory Code assignment?

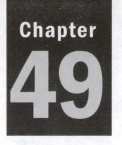
SCAVENGER HUNT

Go to the Justcoding website and ICD-10-PCS Coding quiz: http://www.justcoding.com/quiz/2741

There are five questions to the quiz. How did you do on the quiz the first try? How many times did it take you to get all five questions correct? What are the correct answers for each of the five questions? Of the five questions, which one was the hardest for you to find the correct code, and why?

APPLICATION ASSIGNMENT

Go to AHIMA's website, and read the following article on ICD-10-PCS Root Operation Groups: http://library.ahima.org/xpedio/groups/public/documents/ahima/bok1_046693.hcsp?dDocName=bok1_046693

What did you find most beneficial from this article, and why? As a coder, why is it important to understand the root operations, and what are some ways you will remember the definitions for the 31 root operations?

CRITICAL THINKING

Select one of the Official Coding Guidelines that deals with ICD-10-PCS Coding from those in Table of Contents A: Conventions (the official guidelines can be found at: http://cms.hhs.gov/Medicare/Coding/ICD10/Downloads/2015-PCS-guidelines.pdf).

Describe what the guideline is saying and how we will use this in coding. Give a scenario example of when this guideline would be applied.

CODING CASES

1. Amnioscopy. What is the correct ICD-10-PCS Code assigned?

2. Cystoscopy. What is the correct ICD-10-PCS Code assigned?

3. Hemodialysis. What is the correct ICD-10-PCS Code assigned?

4. Colonoscopy. What is the correct ICD-10-PCS Code assigned?

5. Ambulatory cardiac monitoring. What is the correct ICD-10-PCS Code assigned?

6. Left intraocular telescope. What is the correct ICD-10-PCS Code assigned?

7. Determination of mental status. What is the correct ICD-10-PCS Code assigned?

8. Hypnosis. What is the correct ICD-10-PCS Code assigned?

9. Isolation. What is the correct ICD-10-PCS Code assigned?

10. Aquapheresis. What is the correct ICD-10-PCS Code assigned?

11. Manually assisted delivery. What is the correct ICD-10-PCS Code assigned?

12. Esophagogastroscopy. What is the correct ICD-10-PCS Code assigned?

13. Artificial insemination. What is the correct ICD-10-PCS Code assigned?

14. Crisis intervention. What is the correct ICD-10-PCS Code assigned?

15. Anoscopy. What is the correct ICD-10-PCS Code assigned?

16. Esophagoscopy. What is the correct ICD-10-PCS Code assigned?

17. Intermittent negative airway pressure for 16 hours. What is the correct ICD-10-PCS Code assigned?

18. Detoxification services for substance abuse. What is the correct ICD-10-PCS Code assigned?

19. Choledochoscopy. What is the correct ICD-10-PCS Code assigned?

20. Cardiopulmonary bypass. What is the correct ICD-10-PCS Code assigned?

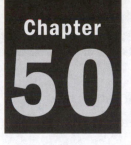

THE STRUCTURE OF MEDICAL AND SURGICAL PROCEDURE CODES

SCAVENGER HUNT

Go to the Justcoding website and ICD-10-PCS Coding quiz: http://www
.justcoding.com/quiz/2093

There are five questions to the quiz. How did you do on the quiz the first
try? How many times did it take you to get all five questions correct? What
are the correct answers for each of the five questions? Of the five questions,
which one was the hardest for you to find the correct code, and why?

APPLICATION ASSIGNMENT

Go to HCPRO's website, and read the blog on ICD-10-PCS: http://blogs
.hcpro.com/icd-10/2010/05/a-code-to-remember/

What did you find most beneficial about this blog? What do you think about
the mnemonic used? Will that help you remember the seven-digit structure
in PCS coding? Why or why not? Have you found something else useful in
remember the characters in PCS codes?

CRITICAL THINKING

Select one of the Official Coding Guidelines that deals with ICD-10-PCS
Coding from those in Table of Contents B.2: Body System (the official
guidelines can be found at http://cms.hhs.gov/Medicare/Coding/ICD10/
Downloads/2015-PCS-guidelines.pdf).

Describe what the guideline is saying and how we will use this in coding.
Give a scenario example of when this guideline would be applied.

CODING CASES

1. Light Therapy. What is the correct ICD-10-PCS Code assigned?
2. Multiple sleep latency test. What is the correct ICD-10-PCS Code
   assigned?
3. Polysomnogram. What is the correct ICD-10-PCS Code assigned?
4. Laryngoscopy. What is the correct ICD-10-PCS Code assigned?
5. Resection of a fingernail. What is the correct ICD-10-PCS Code
   assigned?

6. Narcosynthesis. What is the correct ICD-10-PCS Code assigned?

7. Shirodkar cervical cerclage. What is the correct ICD-10-PCS Code assigned?

8. Impedance phlebography. What is the correct ICD-10-PCS Code assigned?

9. Open cardiac massage. What is the correct ICD-10-PCS Code assigned?

10. Proctoscopy. What is the correct ICD-10-PCS Code assigned?

11. Psychoanalysis. What is the correct ICD-10-PCS Code assigned?

12. Spinal blood patch. What is the correct ICD-10-PCS Code assigned?

13. Pyloroscopy. What is the correct ICD-10-PCS Code assigned?

14. Mediastinoscopy. What is the correct ICD-10-PCS Code assigned?

15. Antabuse pharmacotherapy. What is the correct ICD-10-PCS Code assigned?

16. Pinealoscopy. What is the correct ICD-10-PCS Code assigned?

17. Meditation. What is the correct ICD-10-PCS Code assigned?

18. Therapeutic plasmapheresis. What is the correct ICD-10-PCS Code assigned?

19. Percutaneous endoscopic gastrostomy. What is the correct ICD-10-PCS Code assigned?

20. Medication management. What is the correct ICD-10-PCS Code assigned?

CODING FOR MEDICAL AND SURGICAL PROCEDURES

SCAVENGER HUNT

Go to the Justcoding website and ICD-10-PCS Coding quiz: http://www .justcoding.com/quiz/2595

There are five questions to the quiz. How did you do on the quiz the first try? How many times did it take you to get all five questions correct? What are the correct answers for each of the five questions? Of the five questions, which one was the hardest for you to find the correct code, and why?

APPLICATION ASSIGNMENT

Go to HCPRO's website, and read the following article on getting to know the ICD-10-PCS root operations: http://www.justcoding.com/290935/ get-to-know-the-icd10pcs-root-operations

What did you find most beneficial about this article, and why? Did you find any tips that you can use in your future coding career? What are some ways you will utilize the root operations definitions presented as you prepare for ICD-10-PCS coding?

CRITICAL THINKING

Select one of the Official Coding Guidelines that deals with ICD-10-PCS Coding from those in Table of Contents B.3.1a–B3.5: Root Operation (the official guidelines can be found at http://cms.hhs.gov/Medicare/Coding/ ICD10/Downloads/2015-PCS-guidelines.pdf).

Describe what the guideline is saying and how we will use this in coding. Give a scenario example of when this guideline would be applied.

CODING CASES

1. Transurethral resection of the prostate. What is the correct ICD-10-PCS Code assigned?

2. Left finger transfer. What is the correct ICD-10-PCS Code assigned?

3. Bilateral superficial inferior epigastric artery flap. What is the correct ICD-10-PCS Code assigned?

4. Rhinoscopy. What is the correct ICD-10-PCS Code assigned?

5. Reclosure of disrupted abdominal wall. What is the correct ICD-10-PCS Code assigned?

6. Left lens extraction. What is the correct ICD-10-PCS Code assigned?

7. Percutaneous endoscopic jejunostomy for feeding. What is the correct ICD-10-PCS Code assigned?

8. Reposition of the right nipple. What is the correct ICD-10-PCS Code assigned?

9. Extirpation of the skin of the neck. What is the correct ICD-10-PCS Code assigned?

10. Detachment of left shoulder region. What is the correct ICD-10-PCS Code assigned?

11. Reattachment of the right thumb. What is the correct ICD-10-PCS Code assigned?

12. Insertion of neurostimular generator device in the skull. What is the correct ICD-10-PCS Code assigned?

13. Hair extraction. What is the correct ICD-10-PCS Code assigned?

14. Resection of the right auditory ossicle. What is the correct ICD-10-PCS Code assigned?

15. Umbilical vein catheterization for infusion. What is the correct ICD-10-PCS Code assigned?

16. Destruction of the right sclera. What is the correct ICD-10-PCS Code assigned?

17. Release of the left retinal vessel. What is the correct ICD-10-PCS Code assigned?

18. EGD. What is the correct ICD-10-PCS Code assigned?

19. Extirpation of the left conjunctiva. What is the correct ICD-10-PCS Code assigned?

20. Repair of the skin on the abdomen. What is the correct ICD-10-PCS Code assigned?

CODING PRACTICE

Case 1

Nancy Newhouse is a 55-year-old patient who was recently diagnosed with Stage I carcinoma of her left breast. Nancy is being admitted today for a mastectomy of her left breast. Nancy is taken to the OR, prepped, draped, and anesthetized. An incision is made around the breast, and the breast is removed. The specimen is sent to pathology. What is the correct ICD-10-PCS code assigned?

Case 2

Molly Meanders is brought in today with severe abdominal pain. She had a CT scan done, which revealed a ruptured cyst on her right ovary. Molly has a significant amount of bleeding and is taken to the OR to explore her ovary. An incision was made, and the ovary was visualized. A fragment was seen from a ruptured cyst. The cyst was removed, and the leaking vessel was cauterized. Molly was taken to the recovery room and sent home the next day. What is the correct ICD-10-PCS code assigned?

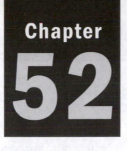

SECTION FOR ROOT
OPERATIONS B, T, 6, 5, D

 ## SCAVENGER HUNT

Go to the Justcoding website and ICD-10-PCS Coding quiz: http://www
.justcoding.com/quiz/1986

There are five questions to the quiz. How did you do on the quiz the first
try? How many times did it take you to get all five questions correct? What
are the correct answers for each of the five questions? Of the five questions,
which one was the hardest for you to find the correct code, and why?

APPLICATION ASSIGNMENT

Go to MedlinePlus, and watch the video on a prostatectomy via the following link: http://www.orlive.com/south-miami-hospital/videos/watch-south-
miami-hospital-surgeons-perform-robot-assisted-prostatectomy?view=display
pageNLM

After you watch the video, what was the most interesting part of it? As a
coder, is it important to visually understand what you are coding? Why or
why not? How do you think this video will be beneficial to you in your future
coding career using ICD-10-PCS codes?

CRITICAL THINKING

Select one of the Official Coding Guidelines that deals with ICD-10-PCS
Coding from those in Table of Contents B.3.6a–B.3.10c: Root Operation
(the official guidelines can be found at http://cms.hhs.gov/Medicare/Coding/
ICD10/Downloads/2015-PCS-guidelines.pdf).

Describe what the guideline is saying and how we will use this in coding.
Give a scenario example of when this guideline would be applied.

CODING CASES

1. Excision of abdominal aorta, open approach. What is the correct ICD-10-PCS Code assigned?

2. Destruction of left hypogastric vein, percutaneous approach. What is the correct ICD-10-PCS Code assigned?

3. Open resection of upper lip. What is the correct ICD-10-PCS Code assigned?

4. Colonoscopy with polypectomy of the descending colon. What is the correct ICD-10-PCS Code assigned?

5. Laryngoscopy with removal of trachea. What is the correct ICD-10-PCS Code assigned?

6. Excision of inferior mesenteric artery, percutaneous approach, diagnostic. What is the correct ICD-10-PCS Code assigned?

7. Fitting of a left leg prosthesis. What is the correct ICD-10-PCS Code assigned?

8. Resection of upper tooth. What is the correct ICD-10-PCS Code assigned?

9. Destruction of liver lesion. What is the correct ICD-10-PCS Code assigned?

10. Removal of the pancreas. What is the correct ICD-10-PCS Code assigned?

11. Excision of left foot artery, open approach, diagnostic. What is the correct ICD-10-PCS Code assigned?

12. Chiropractic manual manipulation of the lumbar spine. What is the correct ICD-10-PCS Code assigned?

13. Duodenectomy. What is the correct ICD-10-PCS Code assigned?

14. Psychoanalysis. What is the correct ICD-10-PCS Code assigned?

15. Destruction of left cephalic vein, open approach. What is the correct ICD-10-PCS Code assigned?

16. Bronchoscopy with removal of left upper bronchial lobe. What is the correct ICD-10-PCS Code assigned?

17. Aquapheresis. What is the correct ICD-10-PCS Code assigned?

18. Esophagoscopy with biopsy of the esophagus. What is the correct ICD-10-PCS Code assigned?

19. Tonsillectomy, What is the correct ICD-10-PCS Code assigned?

20. Open extraction of right brachial vein. What is the correct ICD-10-PCS Code assigned?

CODING PRACTICE

Case 1

Lucas Ludwig is a 17-year-old with abnormal growth concerns, and the physician is concerned about a mass on his pituitary gland. Lucas is brought to the OR, where he is prepped, draped, and given anesthesia. The surgeon makes a 1-cm incision into his neck and visualizes the pituitary gland. The mass is on the superior portion, which was excised and sent to pathology for review. What is the correct ICD-10-PCS code assigned?

Case 2

Ava Airhart is a 5-day-old infant who is admitted for severe jaundice. Ava is given phototherapy to her chest three times a day for 60 minutes each time for 2 days, and the jaundice is improved. Ava is discharged to home with instructions to follow up if the jaundice reappears. What is the correct ICD-10-PCS code assigned?

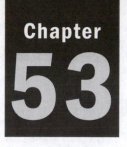
SECTION O ROOT
OPERATIONS Y, M, X, S

SCAVENGER HUNT

Go to the Justcoding website and ICD-10-PCS Coding quiz: http://www
.justcoding.com/quiz/2839

There are five questions to the quiz. How did you do on the quiz the first
try? How many times did it take you to get all five questions correct?
What are the correct answers for each of the five questions? Of the five
questions, which one was the hardest for you to find the correct code,
and why?

APPLICATION ASSIGNMENT

Go to MedlinePlus, and watch the video of a fracture repair via
the following link: http://ortho.broadcastmed.com/4120/videos/
surgical-repair-of-a-jones-fracture?view=displayPageNLM

After you watch the video, what was the most interesting part of it? As a
coder, is it important to visually understand what you are coding? Why or
why not? How do you think this video will be beneficial to you in your future
coding career using ICD-10-PCS codes?

CRITICAL THINKING

Select one of the Official Coding Guidelines that deals with ICD-10-PCS
Coding from those in Table of Contents B.3.11a–B.3.16: Root Operation
(the official guidelines can be found at http://cms.hhs.gov/Medicare/Coding/
ICD10/Downloads/2015-PCS-guidelines.pdf).

Describe what the guideline is saying and how we will use this in coding.
Give a scenario example of when this guideline would be applied.

CODING CASES

1. Open transfer of the olfactory nerve to the hypoglossal nerve. What is the correct ICD-10-PCS Code assigned?

2. Open allogeneic heart transplantation. What is the correct ICD-10-PCS Code assigned?

3. Reposition of the thoracic aorta. What is the correct ICD-10-PCS Code assigned?

4. Closed reduction of a dislocation of the left shoulder. What is the correct ICD-10-PCS Code assigned?

5. Reattachment of left cheek. What is the correct ICD-10-PCS Code assigned?

6. Open with reposition of the right spermatic cord. What is the correct ICD-10-PCS Code assigned?

7. Open repositioning of the thoracic spinal cord. What is the correct ICD-10-PCS Code assigned?

8. Hysteroscopy with reposition of the right fallopian tube. What is the correct ICD-10-PCS Code assigned?

9. Repositioning of the urethra. What is the correct ICD-10-PCS Code assigned?

10. Closed reduction of right finer phalangeal joint dislocation. What is the correct ICD-10-PCS Code assigned?

11. Reattachment of the penis. What is the correct ICD-10-PCS Code assigned?

12. An incision was made, and the deltoid muscle from the left shoulder was reattached after it was ripped during a motorcycle accident. What is the correct ICD-10-PCS Code assigned?

13. Open reduction of left upper femur fracture. Four intramedullary nails were implanted. What is the correct ICD-10-PCS Code assigned?

14. Transplantation of syngeneic left ovary. What is the correct ICD-10-PCS Code assigned?

15. Arthroscopy with transfer of the radial nerve to the median nerve. What is the correct ICD-10-PCS Code assigned?

16. Reattachment of left lower arm. What is the correct ICD-10-PCS Code assigned?

17. Open transfer of left index finger to left thumb. What is the correct ICD-10-PCS Code assigned?

18. ORIF left wrist joint. What is the correct ICD-10-PCS Code assigned?

19. Liver transplant from donor matched liver. What is the correct ICD-10-PCS Code assigned?

20. Percutaneous repositioning of the sciatic nerve. What is the correct ICD-10-PCS Code assigned?

CODING PRACTICE

Case 1

Steven Small is a patient who has been on hemodialysis with end-stage renal failure awaiting a kidney transplant. Today he is admitted for the kidney transplant as a donor was identified and the kidney was received. The patient is taken to the OR, prepped, draped, and anesthetized. A kidney transplant on the right side is completed without any complications. What is the correct ICD-10-PCS code assigned?

Case 2

Christopher Callhoun was involved in an accident on his farm, and the nerves in his left hand were compromised. He is brought to surgery today for a nerve transfer to help restore function in his left hand. The patient is prepped, draped, and anesthetized. An incision is made over the patient's left hand where the median nerve is grafted to the ulnar nerve using an operating microscope. What is the correct ICD-10-PCS code assigned?

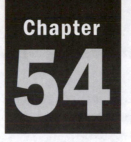
SECTION O ROOT
OPERATIONS V, L, 7, 1

SCAVENGER HUNT

Go to the Justcoding website and ICD-10-PCS Coding quiz: http://www
.justcoding.com/quiz/2787

There are five questions to the quiz. How did you do on the quiz the first
try? How many times did it take you to get all five questions correct? What
are the correct answers for each of the five questions? Of the five questions,
which one was the hardest for you to find the correct code, and why?

APPLICATION ASSIGNMENT

Go to MedlinePlus, and watch the video of an aortic valve bypass surgery via the following link: http://cardiac.broadcastmed.com/3979/videos/
aortic-valve-bypass-surgery?view=displayPageNLM

After you watch the video, what was the most interesting part of it? As a
coder, is it important to visually understand what you are coding? Why or
why not? How do you think this video will be beneficial to you in your future
coding career using ICD-10-PCS codes?

CRITICAL THINKING

Select one of the Official Coding Guidelines that deals with ICD-10-
PCS Coding from those in Table of Contents B.4: Body Part (the official
guidelines can be found at http://cms.hhs.gov/Medicare/Coding/ICD10/
Downloads/2015-PCS-guidelines.pdf).

Describe what the guideline is saying and how we will use this in coding.
Give a scenario example of when this guideline would be applied.

CODING CASES

1. CABG x2 was performed using the thoracic artery. What is the correct
   ICD-10-PCS Code assigned?

2. Open restriction of the right subclavian artery. What is the correct
   ICD-10-PCS Code assigned?

3. Percutaneous occlusion of right pulmonary vein. What is the correct
   ICD-10-PCS Code assigned?

4. An incision was made over the brachial artery, and a bypass of left brachial artery to left upper arm artery was completed. What is the correct ICD-10-PCS Code assigned?

5. Endoscopic Roux-en-Y esophageal bypass with anastomosis to the duodenum. What is the correct ICD-10-PCS Code assigned?

6. Single treatment of hemodialysis. What is the correct ICD-10-PCS Code assigned?

7. Application of compression dressing to the back. What is the correct ICD-10-PCS Code assigned?

8. Open bypass of the esophageal vein to lower vein using a synthetic substitute. What is the correct ICD-10-PCS Code assigned?

9. Cystoscopy with intraluminal dilation of a stricture in the neck of the bladder. What is the correct ICD-10-PCS Code assigned?

10. Ventridculocisternostomy from the 3rd ventricle to the cisterna magna using an autologous tissue substitute. What is the correct ICD-10-PCS Code assigned?

11. Percutaneous irrigation of the spinal canal using an irrigating substance. What is the correct ICD-10-PCS Code assigned?

12. Reattachment of the skin to the left ear. What is the correct ICD-10-PCS Code assigned?

13. Endoscopy with occlusion of the common bile duct using an intraluminal device. What is the correct ICD-10-PCS Code assigned?

14. Right hemicolectomy was performed with formation of transverse colon colostomy. What is the correct ICD-10-PCS Code assigned?

15. An incision was made over the right hand and a reattachment of the right hand tendon was completed. What is the correct ICD-10-PCS Code assigned?

16. Laparoscopic bilateral fallopian tube ligation. What is the correct ICD-10-PCS Code assigned?

17. Percutaneous irrigation of the peritoneal cavity using dialysate. What is the correct ICD-10-PCS Code assigned?

18. Upper endoscopy with balloon dilation of the esophagus. What is the correct ICD-10-PCS Code assigned?

19. Open dilation of right internal mammary artery with drug-eluting stent. What is the correct ICD-10-PCS Code assigned?

20. PTCA of three coronary arteries with insertion of drug-eluting stents. What is the correct ICD-10-PCS Code assigned?

CODING PRACTICE

Case 1

Genevieve Gester has a solitary fallopian tube and is admitted today for ligation of this tube. An incision was made, and the endoscope was inserted. An endoscopic ligation of the right fallopian tube using a fallopian ring was performed. What is the correct ICD-10-PCS code assigned?

Case 2

Sixty-five-year-old Sandy Sampson has Stage 3 adenocarcinoma of the colon. The tumor was resected previously, and now Sandy is being admitted for a bypass with formation of a colostomy. Sandy is taken to the OR, prepped, draped, and anesthetized. Her previous incision is reopened, and the sigmoid colon is taken to the rectum, where a colostomy was created. What is the correct ICD-10-PCS code assigned?

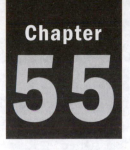
SECTION 0 ROOT
OPERATIONS 9, C, F, N, 8, J, K

SCAVENGER HUNT

Go to the Justcoding website and ICD-10-PCS Coding quiz: http://www
.justcoding.com/quiz/2051

There are five questions to the quiz. How did you do on the quiz the first
try? How many times did it take you to get all five questions correct? What
are the correct answers for each of the five questions? Of the five questions,
which one was the hardest for you to find the correct code, and why?

APPLICATION ASSIGNMENT

Go to MedlinePlus, and watch the video of a lithotripsy via the
following link: http://www.orlive.com/broward-health/videos/
kidney-stone-treatment-with-lithotripsy?view=displayPageNLM

After you watch the video, what was the most interesting part of it? As a
coder, is it important to visually understand what you are coding? Why or
why not? How do you think this video will be beneficial to you in your future
coding career using ICD-10-PCS codes?

CRITICAL THINKING

Select one of the Official Coding Guidelines that deals with ICD-10-
PCS Coding from those in Table of Contents 5: Approach (the official
guidelines can be found at http://cms.hhs.gov/Medicare/Coding/ICD10/
Downloads/2015-PCS-guidelines.pdf).

Describe what the guideline is saying and how we will use this in coding.
Give a scenario example of when this guideline would be applied.

CODING CASES

1. Percutaneous thrombectomy of right brachial artery. What is the cor-
    rect ICD-10-PCS Code assigned?

2. Antrostomy of the right middle ear. What is the correct ICD-10-PCS
    Code assigned?

3. Choledochoscopy. What is the correct ICD-10-PCS Code assigned?

4. Cystotomy with percutaneous drainage of the bladder. What is the correct ICD-10-PCS Code assigned?

5. Open arthrolysis of the right elbow joint. What is the correct ICD-10-PCS Code assigned?

6. Drainage of the buccal mucosa via external drainage tube. What is the correct ICD-10-PCS Code assigned?

7. Percutaneous gastrotomy. What is the correct ICD-10-PCS Code assigned?

8. Arthrocentesis of effusion via needle in the right acromioclavicular joint. What is the correct ICD-10-PCS Code assigned?

9. Laparotomy with inspection of abdominal wall. What is the correct ICD-10-PCS Code assigned?

10. Gastroscopy with stomach release. What is the correct ICD-10-PCS Code assigned?

11. Arthroscopy of the cervical vertebral disc. What is the correct ICD-10-PCS Code assigned?

12. Open extirpation of cervical vertebral disc. What is the correct ICD-10-PCS Code assigned?

13. Duodenoscopy with duodenolysis. What is the correct ICD-10-PCS Code assigned?

14. Drainage of the right vitreous. What is the correct ICD-10-PCS Code assigned?

15. Laparoscopic inspection of the gallbladder. What is the correct ICD-10-PCS Code assigned?

16. Hysteroscopy. What is the correct ICD-10-PCS Code assigned?

17. Exploratory laparotomy with inspection of the pelvic cavity. What is the correct ICD-10-PCS Code assigned?

18. Endoscopic endarterectomy of the right common carotid artery. What is the correct ICD-10-PCS Code assigned?

19. Esophageal release. What is the correct ICD-10-PCS Code assigned?

20. Thoracotomy of chest wall. What is the correct ICD-10-PCS Code assigned?

CODING PRACTICE

Case 1

A 17-year-old was admitted today from life flight after a rollover collision in which he was the driver. He had a collapsed lung and was taken to the OR for an emergency thoracostomy to repair his left collapsed lung. What is the correct ICD-10-PCS code assigned?

Case 2

A 4-year-old with an abscess on her left adenoid. She is brought to the OR, where she is prepped, draped, and given anesthesia. Her left adenoid is visualized, and an incision is made to drain the abscess. What is the correct ICD-10-PCS code assigned?

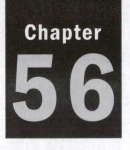

SECTION O ROOT OPERATIONS
H, R, U, 2, P, W, 3, Q, G, O, 4

SCAVENGER HUNT

Go to the Justcoding website and ICD-10-PCS Coding quiz: http://www.justcoding.com/quiz/2911

There are five questions to the quiz. How did you do on the quiz the first try? How many times did it take you to get all five questions correct? What are the correct answers for each of the five questions? Of the five questions, which one was the hardest for you to find the correct code, and why?

APPLICATION ASSIGNMENT

Go to MedlinePlus, and watch the video of a spinal fusion via the following link: http://ortho.broadcastmed.com/4033/videos/spinal-fusion-surgery-for-relief-of-chronic-lower-back-pain?view=displayPageNLM

After you watch the video, what was the most interesting part of it? As a coder, is it important to visually understand what you are coding? Why or why not? How do you think this video will be beneficial to you in your future coding career using ICD-10-PCS codes?

CRITICAL THINKING

Select one of the Official Coding Guidelines that deals with ICD-10-PCS Coding from those in Table of Contents B.6: Device (the official guidelines can be found at http://cms.hhs.gov/Medicare/Coding/ICD10/Downloads/2015-PCS-guidelines.pdf).

Describe what the guideline is saying and how we will use this in coding. Give a scenario example of when this guideline would be applied.

CODING CASES

1. Total knee replacement with a polyethylene implant of the right knee. What is the correct ICD-10-PCS Code assigned?

2. Open arthrodesis of the left ankle. What is the correct ICD-10-PCS Code assigned?

3. Left finger phalangeal joint replacement with prosthetic implant. What is the correct ICD-10-PCS Code assigned?

4. Repair of an upper lip cleft lip. What is the correct ICD-10-PCS Code assigned?

5. Dual-chamber cardiac pacemaker lead revision. What is the correct ICD-10-PCS Code assigned?

6. Open heart repair of the mitral valve. What is the correct ICD-10-PCS Code assigned?

7. Insertion of an infusion device into the Thymus. What is the correct ICD-10-PCS Code assigned?

8. Open repair of right inguinal hernia with mesh. What is the correct ICD-10-PCS Code assigned?

9. Radical bilateral mastectomy with insertion of a tissue expander. What is the correct ICD-10-PCS Code assigned?

10. Arthroscopy with arthrodesis of the right carpal joint. What is the correct ICD-10-PCS Code assigned?

11. External revision of drainage device in urethra. What is the correct ICD-10-PCS Code assigned?

12. Open repair of the olfactory nerve. What is the correct ICD-10-PCS Code assigned?

13. Right shoulder arthroplasty with autologous tissue substitute. What is the correct ICD-10-PCS Code assigned?

14. Open arytenoidopexy of the larynx. What is the correct ICD-10-PCS Code assigned?

15. External balanoplasty. What is the correct ICD-10-PCS Code assigned?

16. Change in drainage device from abdominal wall. What is the correct ICD-10-PCS Code assigned?

17. Septoplasty with repair of septal deviation was performed. What is the correct ICD-10-PCS Code assigned?

18. Open repair of the thoracic spinal cord. What is the correct ICD-10-PCS Code assigned?

19. Valvuloplasty with replacement of the pulmonary valve with a bovine valve. What is the correct ICD-10-PCS Code assigned?

20. Open repair of the left acromioclavicular joint. What is the correct ICD-10-PCS Code assigned?

CODING PRACTICE

Case 1

Sixty-seven-year-old Maggie Millcreek has severe osteoarthritis in her left hip. She is admitted today for a total hip replacement of her left hip. She was taken to the OR, prepped, draped, and anesthetized. An incision was made over her left hip, and the hip was removed and replaced with a ceramic synthetic substitute that was cemented in. What is the correct ICD-10-PCS code assigned?

Case 2

A 34-year-old was seen today for a mastorrhaphy of the left breast. She was brought to the OR, where she was prepped, draped, and given anesthesia. An incision was made over the defective tissue of the left breast, and a mastorrhaphy was completed without any complications. What is the correct ICD-10-PCS code assigned?

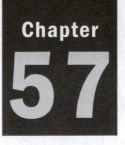

MEDICAL AND SURGICAL-RELATED PROCEDURES

SCAVENGER HUNT

Go to the Justcoding website and ICD-10-PCS Coding quiz: http://www
.justcoding.com/quiz/2762

There are five questions to the quiz. How did you do on the quiz the first
try? How many times did it take you to get all five questions correct?
What are the correct answers for each of the five questions? Of the five
questions, which one was the hardest for you to find the correct code,
and why?

APPLICATION ASSIGNMENT

Go to MedlinePlus, and watch the video of radiation therapy via the following link: http://www.orlive.com/hartfordhospital/videos/trilogy-stereotactic-
radiation-therapy-for-brain-tumors1?view=displayPageNLM

After you watch the video, what was the most interesting part of it? As a
coder, is it important to visually understand what you are coding? Why or
why not? How do you think this video will be beneficial to you in your future
coding career using ICD-10-PCS codes?

CRITICAL THINKING

Select one of the Official Coding Guidelines that deals with ICD-10-
PCS Coding from those in Table of Contents C: Obstetrics (the official
guidelines can be found at http://cms.hhs.gov/Medicare/Coding/ICD10/
Downloads/2015-PCS-guidelines.pdf).

Describe what the guideline is saying and how we will use this in coding.
Give a scenario example of when this guideline would be applied.

CODING CASES

1. Diagnostic amniocentesis. What is the correct ICD-10-PCS Code assigned?

2. Induction of labor with oxytocin. What is the correct ICD-10-PCS Code assigned?

3. Vacuum-assisted delivery of healthy liveborn male infant. What is the correct ICD-10-PCS Code assigned?

4. Delivery complicated by large infant and the use of low forceps were utilized. What is the correct ICD-10-PCS Code assigned?

5. Fetal scalp electrode was changed to monitor fetal heart rate. What is the correct ICD-10-PCS Code assigned?

6. Patient seen to have the right foot brace changed. What is the correct ICD-10-PCS Code assigned?

7. Peritoneal dialysis. What is the correct ICD-10-PCS Code assigned?

8. Neck traction. What is the correct ICD-10-PCS Code assigned?

9. Change in splint on right thumb. What is the correct ICD-10-PCS Code assigned?

10. Hemodialysis. What is the correct ICD-10-PCS Code assigned?

11. Change in the packing material from anorectal fistula repair. What is the correct ICD-10-PCS Code assigned?

12. Removal of packing material from left ear. What is the correct ICD-10-PCS Code assigned?

13. Low transverse cervical C-section delivery. What is the correct ICD-10-PCS Code assigned?

14. Packing material changed in the abdominal wall. What is the correct ICD-10-PCS Code assigned?

15. Insertion of packing in left ear. What is the correct ICD-10-PCS Code assigned?

16. Chiropractic manipulation of the sacrum. What is the correct ICD-10-PCS Code assigned?

17. Removal of nasal packing. What is the correct ICD-10-PCS Code assigned?

18. Breech presentation of fetus so an external rotation was performed to aid in the vaginal delivery of the infant. What is the correct ICD-10-PCS Code assigned?

19. Manually assisted spontaneous delivery. What is the correct ICD-10-PCS Code assigned?

20. Vaginal transplantation of products of conception. What is the correct ICD-10-PCS Code assigned?

CODING PRACTICE

Case 1

A 16-year-old with an unwanted pregnancy is admitted today for an abortion. A speculum was inserted into the vagina, and a vacuum was used to complete the vaginal abortion at 8-weeks gestation. What is the correct ICD-10-PCS Code assigned?

Case 2

A 27-year-old female in active labor with contractions 5 minutes apart is admitted. The physician comes in to check the progress of the patient and performs an artificial rupture of membranes to progress her labor. What is the correct ICD-10-PCS Code assigned?

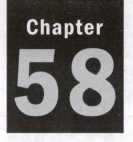

ANCILLARY PROCEDURES

SCAVENGER HUNT

Go to the Justcoding website and ICD-10-PCS Coding quiz: http://www .justcoding.com/quiz/2227

There are five questions to the quiz. How did you do on the quiz the first try? How many times did it take you to get all five questions correct? What are the correct answers for each of the five questions? Of the five questions, which one was the hardest for you to find the correct code, and why?

APPLICATION ASSIGNMENT

Go to MedlinePlus, and watch the video of a hearing procedure via the following link: http://www.orlive.com/hartfordhospital/videos/ baha-bone-anchored-hearing-treatment-procedure2?view=displayPageNLM

After you watch the video, what was the most interesting part of it? As a coder, is it important to visually understand what you are coding? Why or why not? How do you think this video will be beneficial to you in your future coding career using ICD-10-PCS codes?

CRITICAL THINKING

Select one of the Official Coding Guidelines that deals with ICD-10-PCS Coding from those in Table of Contents D: Selection of Principal Diagnosis (the official guidelines can be found at http://cms.hhs.gov/Medicare/Coding/ ICD10/Downloads/2015-PCS-guidelines.pdf).

Describe what the guideline is saying and how we will use this in coding. Give a scenario example of when this guideline would be applied.

CODING CASES

1. Bilateral carotid artery ultrasound. What is the correct ICD-10-PCS Code assigned?

2. Electroconvulsive therapy. What is the correct ICD-10-PCS Code assigned?

3. High osmolar fluoroscopy of the spine. What is the correct ICD-10-PCS Code assigned?

4. Gait training with a walker. What is the correct ICD-10-PCS Code assigned?

5. Hearing screening with a tympanometer. What is the correct ICD-10-PCS Code assigned?

6. Twelve-step group counseling. What is the correct ICD-10-PCS Code assigned?

7. Hyperthermia, radiation therapy of the chest. What is the correct ICD-10-PCS Code assigned?

8. CT of the abdomen and pelvis with low osmolar contrast. What is the correct ICD-10-PCS Code assigned?

9. Group psychotherapy. What is the correct ICD-10-PCS Code assigned?

10. MRI of the right hip. What is the correct ICD-10-PCS Code assigned?

11. Whole body radiography on a 3-day old newborn. What is the correct ICD-10-PCS Code assigned?

12. Ultrasound of the right ovary for evaluation of a cyst. What is the correct ICD-10-PCS Code assigned?

13. Adjustment of patient's Clonidine prescription. What is the correct ICD-10-PCS Code assigned?

14. Nonimaging nuclear medicine probe of the spine. What is the correct ICD-10-PCS Code assigned?

15. Upper airway fluroscopy. What is the correct ICD-10-PCS Code assigned?

16. Enhanced MRI of the brain with contrast. What is the correct ICD-10-PCS Code assigned?

17. Stereotactic radiosurgery via gamma beam to the bladder. What is the correct ICD-10-PCS Code assigned?

18. Patient had a stroke and is now undergoing a bedside swallowing function assessment before he is allowed to eat. What is the correct ICD-10-PCS Code assigned?

19. Methadone Maintenance. What is the correct ICD-10-PCS Code assigned?

20. Ultrasound of the penis. What is the correct ICD-10-PCS Code assigned?

CODING PRACTICE

Case 1

Samuel Smith is seen today by Physical therapy. The physical therapist completed an evaluation to assess his motor function and coordination of both his legs. What is the correct ICD-10-PCS code assigned?

Case 2

Chariot Chymson has breast cancer of her left breast. She is brought into for radiation therapy. Chariot receives brachytherapy to her left breast. The brachytherapy was a low dose rate with I-125 Isotope. She did not experience any problems during the radiation and will return in 1 week. What is the correct ICD-10-PCS code assigned?